Cardiology
explained

Remedica explained series

ISSN 1472-4138

Also available
Anal and rectal diseases explained
Interventional radiology explained

Forthcoming
Common spinal disorders explained

Published by Remedica
32–38 Osnaburgh Street, London, NW1 3ND, UK
Civic Opera Building, 20 North Wacker Drive, Suite 1642, Chicago, IL 60606, USA

Email: info@remedicabooks.com
www.remedicabooks.com

Publisher: Andrew Ward
In-house editors: Tonya Berthoud, Helen James, Roisin O'Brien, & Cath Harris
Design: AS&K Skylight Creative Services

© 2004 Remedica

While every effort is made by the publisher to see that no inaccurate or misleading data, opinions, or statements appear in this book, they wish to make it clear that the material contained in the publication represents a summary of the independent evaluations and opinions of the authors. As a consequence, the authors, publisher, and any sponsoring company accept no responsibility for the consequences of any inaccurate or misleading data or statements. Neither do they endorse the content of the publication or the use of any drug or device in a way that lies outside its current licensed application in any territory.

All rights reserved. No part of this publication may be reproduced, stored in a retrieval system or transmitted in any form or by any means, electronic, mechanical, photocopying, recording or otherwise, without the prior permission of the publisher.

Remedica is a member of the AS&K Media Partnership.

ISBN 1 901346 22 6
British Library Cataloguing-in-Publication Data
A catalogue record for this book is available from the British Library.

Cardiology explained

Euan A Ashley and Josef Niebauer

Euan A Ashley
Division of Cardiovascular Medicine
Stanford University School of Medicine
Falk CVRC, 300 Pasteur Drive
Palo Alto, California 94305
USA

Josef Niebauer
Privatdozent and Consultant Cardiologist
Department of Internal Medicine and Cardiology
University of Leipzig – Heart Center
Strümpellstr. 39
04289 Leipzig
Germany

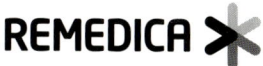

Foreword

Cardiology is a rapidly changing field. New technologies such as drug-eluting stents, left ventricular assist devices, and novel inflammatory markers, and imaging modalities such as magnetic resonance imaging and three-dimensional echocardiography, offer us an unprecedented view of the function of the heart in health and an unparalleled scope of therapies with which to treat disease. Yet, although we cardiologists like to think that we are more innovative and pioneering than our colleagues in other specialties, it seems at least possible that there are equally exciting changes in other fields, too. All of this leaves the generalist as the patient's primary advocate, as the integrator of all these specialist opinions, trying at once to learn enough of the new advances to communicate with both patient and specialist, but not so much as to lose the big picture in amongst the details.

What the generalist needs is a concise, well written, beautifully illustrated guide to cardiology. And fortunately, if you're reading this, you've already found it! The authors have recognized that generalists need help in staying up-to-date with specialist advances in a way that journals can rarely provide: a comprehensive, yet highly digestible update to cardiology that can jog the memory in a tactful but not patronizing way. Further, it is organized not in the didactic way in which many such textbooks are written, but in a way that will make sense to the practicing clinician who needs the facts quickly to hand. Clear yet detailed explanations of what cardiologists do can be found within these pages. Specific guides to understanding cardiological tests and writing good referral letters are two of the unusual, yet extremely useful places where this book differs from others you might have read. All recommendations are, of course, consistent with the latest guidelines from the European Society of Cardiology, the American Heart Association, and the American College of Cardiology. Meanwhile, the historical nuggets remind us from where we have come and just how lucky we are to make it this far (intact!). Together, these things serve to make this book a unique and invaluable resource for generalists and other subspecialists, both in hospital and in the community. I highly commend you for picking it up!

Alan Yeung
Professor of Medicine (Cardiovascular),
Stanford University Medical Center, USA

Preface

We may not be the most impartial commentators, but it seems to us that the heart is the most interesting organ in the body. It beats in a tightly regulated, finely coordinated, gracefully rhythmic fashion to distribute blood and oxygen to all the other organs. It does this more than 2 billion times in the lifetime of an average human. It can accelerate to power an Olympic athlete for 26 miles in a little over 2 hours, and it can weaken to hold your 86-year-old patient hostage in her favorite chair.

Yet the heart, so central to the metaphors of our language, has not revealed its secrets readily. This may be because until relatively recently, it was believed the heart was the only organ that could not be cut (heart surgery was unthinkable from the time of Aristotle until the late 1800s). But this reflects the heart's eternal mystique. Since the invention of the stethoscope we have used technology to reveal the innermost workings of the heart. In recent times, technological advance has been ever more rapid. Indeed, the rapidity of this technological advance is what led us to writing this book. Meanwhile, the bulk of cardiovascular disease remains the realm of the generalists. From whose perspective, knowing when to make use of specialists and knowing how to view their input in the context of the whole patient is increasingly important, yet increasingly difficult. So this is the aim of our book: to sit beside you when you wonder, "Should I refer this patient to a cardiologist"; to look over your shoulder when you receive the cardiology clinic letter; to whisper in your ear the normal left ventricular internal diameter. In short, if our book can be your partner in working with your cardiologist then it has been successful. If it can answer questions the answers to which you once knew, it has been valuable. If it can explain the answers to questions you didn't know you wanted to ask, then it has been worth our while and worth your money. We care deeply that this book fulfils your needs and welcome any feedback on its content, explanatory style, or level of detail.

Many people have made this book possible. Too many to mention in these pages. We would like to thank our wives Fiona and Dörte who have been patient and understanding during the long nights and early mornings. Many cardiologists and generalists gave advice and read chapters and we would like to thank them all here. Finally, we'd like to thank Cath Harris, Andrew Ward, and all the team at Remedica who coaxed and cajoled us, encouraged and enlivened our text, and heroically rescued our diagrams from obscurity.

Euan A Ashley and Josef Niebauer

To Angus Ashley, the best doctor I know

EAA

"To study disease without books is to sail an uncharted sea, while to study books without patients is not to go to sea at all."
William Osler, 1901

"As a cardiologist, I may panic when I see somebody bleed from his nose, but not when I see a heart fibrillate. This is my territory."
Lofty L Basta, 1996

Contents

Chapter 1	Cardiac arrest	1
Chapter 2	Cardiovascular examination	5
Chapter 3	Conquering the ECG	15
Chapter 4	Understanding the echocardiogram	35
Chapter 5	Coronary artery disease	45
Chapter 6	Hypertension	77
Chapter 7	Heart failure	93
Chapter 8	Arrhythmia	111
Chapter 9	Valve disease	145
Chapter 10	Infective endocarditis	167
Chapter 11	Cardiomyopathy	181
Chapter 12	Aneurysm and dissection of the aorta	189
Chapter 13	Pericardial disease	197
Chapter 14	Adult congenital heart disease	203
Abbreviations		215
Index		219

Chapter 1

Cardiac arrest

Adult basic life-support algorithm

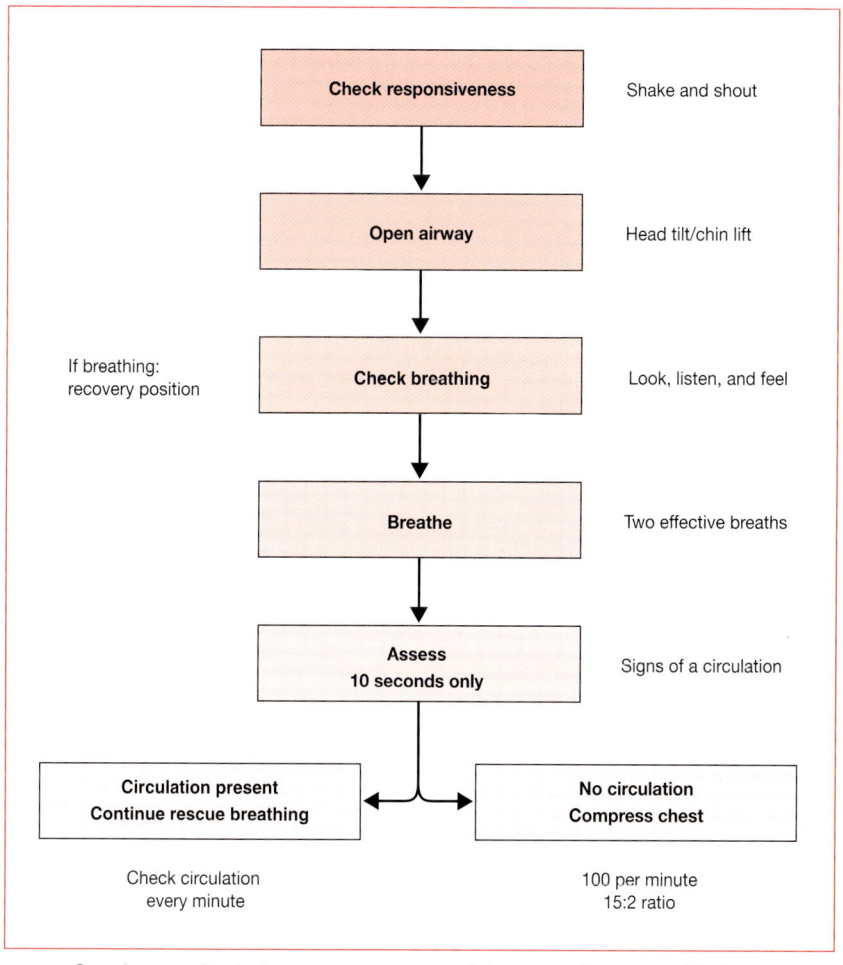

Send or go for help as soon as possible according to guidelines

Chapter 1

Advanced life-support algorithm for the management of cardiac arrest in adults (US version)

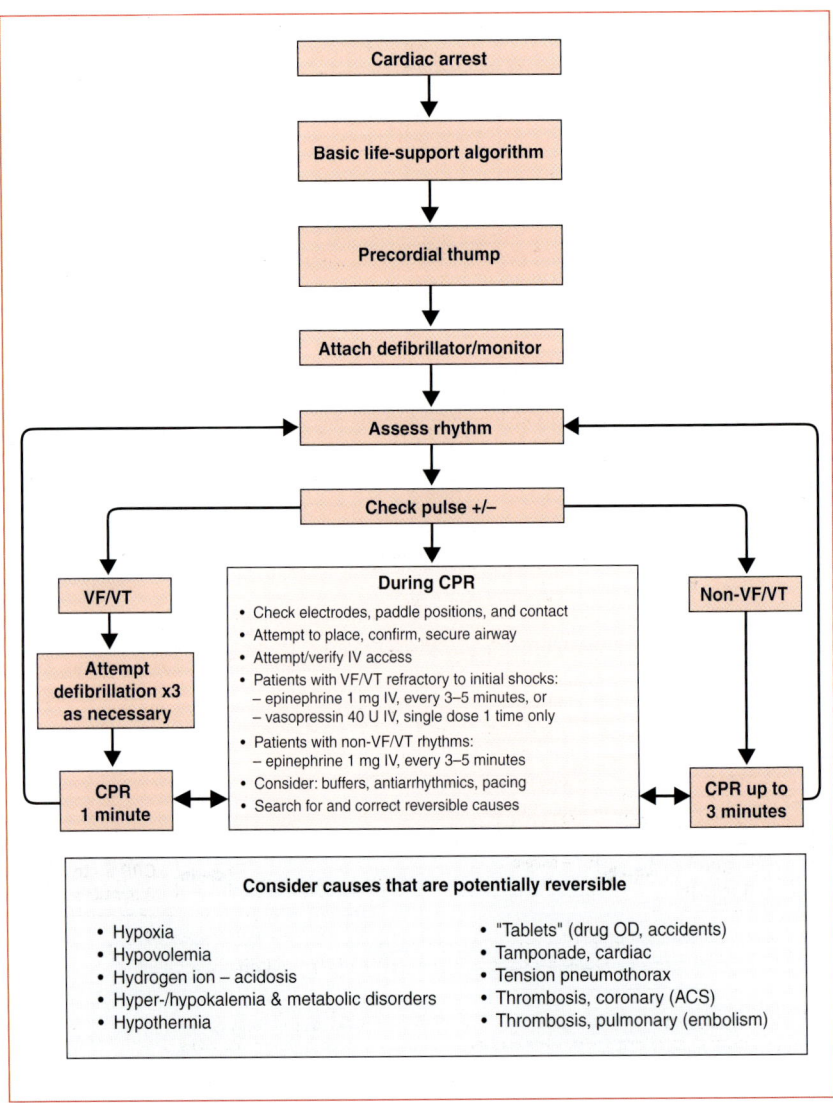

ACS: acute coronary syndromes; CPR: cardiopulmonary resuscitation; IV: intravenous; OD: overdose; VF: ventricular fibrillation; VT: ventricular tachycardia.

Advanced life-support algorithm for the management of cardiac arrest in adults (UK version)

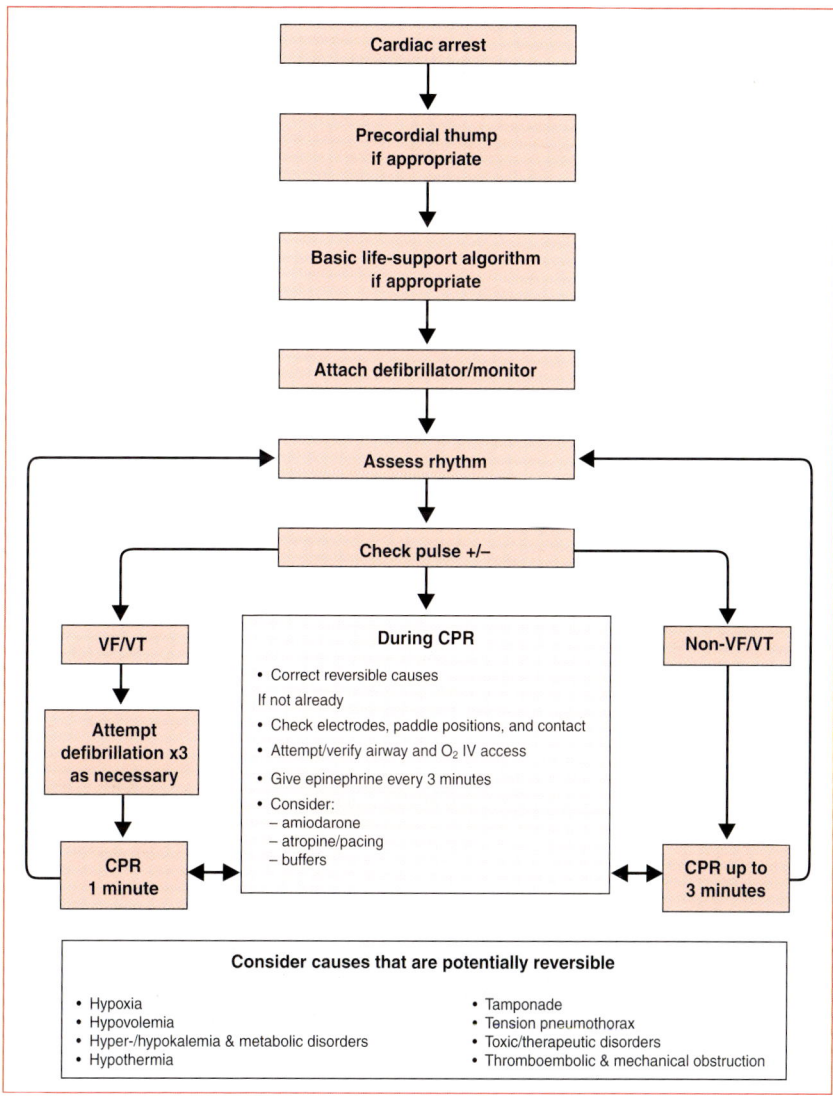

Chapter 1

The adult basic life-support algorithm (UK version) is reprinted with permission from the Resuscitation Council (UK) website and is available at: www.resus.org.uk

The advanced life-support algorithm for the management of cardiac arrest in adults (US version) is reprinted with permission from the American Heart Association (*Circulation* 2000;102:I-143).

The advanced life-support algorithm for the management of cardiac arrest in adults (UK version) is reprinted with permission from the Resuscitation Council (UK) website and is available at: www.resus.org.uk

Chapter 2

Cardiovascular examination

Although technology has a high profile in cardiology, clinical examination remains a central tool, especially for the generalist.

General inspection

Many clues to the cardiac condition can be detected with a simple visual inspection. In the acutely unwell patient, cyanosis, pallor, and sweatiness can all be signs of impending danger – does the patient "look" ill? In nonacute patients, cachexia is perhaps the most important feature to note on general inspection since it is an important prognostic sign in heart failure. Palpation is essential to confirm that girth is excess fluid (pitting edema). Certain physical appearances should always prompt an awareness of cardiac abnormalities (see **Table 1**). Facial signs for which there is evidence of an association with cardiac conditions are shown in **Table 2**. Finally, it is important to document the condition of a potential cardiac patient's teeth.

Genetic disorder	Associated cardiac manifestation
Marfan's syndrome	Aortic regurgitation (aortic dissection)
Down's syndrome	ASD, VSD
Turner's syndrome	Coarctation of the aorta
Spondyloarthritides, eg, ankylosing spondylitis	Aortic regurgitation

Table 1. Cardiac manifestations of genetic disorders. ASD: atrial septal defect; VSD: ventricular septal defect.

Taking the pulse

Taking the pulse is one of the simplest, oldest, and yet most informative of all clinical tests. As you pick up the patient's hand, you should check for clubbing and any peripheral signs of endocarditis (see **Table 3**). Note the rate and document the rhythm of the pulse. The character and volume of the pulse can also be useful signs and traditionally it is believed that these are easier to detect in larger arteries such as the brachial and the carotid (see **Table 4**).

Facial sign	Description	Possible cardiac association
Malar flush	Redness around the cheeks	Mitral stenosis
Xanthomata	Yellowish deposits of lipid around the eyes, palms, or tendons	Hyperlipidemia
Corneal arcus	A ring around the cornea	Age, hyperlipidemia
Proptosis	Forward projection or displacement of the eyeball; occurs in patients with Graves' disease	Atrial fibrillation

Table 2. Facial signs associated with cardiac conditions.

Peripheral sign	Description	Cardiac association
Clubbing	Broadening or thickening of the tips of the fingers (and toes) with increased lengthwise curvature of the nail and a decrease in the angle normally seen between the cuticle and the fingernail	Infective endocarditis, cyanotic congenital heart disease
Splinter hemorrhages	Streak hemorrhages in nailbeds	Infective endocarditis
Janeway lesions	Macules on the back of the hand	Infective endocarditis
Osler's nodes	Tender nodules in fingertips	Infective endocarditis

Table 3. Peripheral signs associated with infective endocarditis.

Checking both radials simultaneously is important in all cases of chest pain as a gross screening test for aortic dissection. Adding radiofemoral delay (or radiofemoral difference in volume) may alert you to coarctation as a rare cause of hypertension.

Peripheral pulses should also be documented, as peripheral vascular disease is an important predictor of coronary artery disease:

- femoral – feel at the midinguinal point (midway between the symphysis pubis and the anterior superior iliac spine, just inferior to the inguinal ligament)
- popliteal – feel deep in the center of the popliteal fossa with the patient lying on their back with their knees bent
- posterior tibial – feel behind the medial malleolus
- dorsalis pedis – feel over the second metatarsal bone just lateral to the extensor hallucis tendon

Cardiovascular examination

Type of pulse	Pulse characteristics	Most likely cause
Regularly irregular	–	2nd-degree heart block, ventricular bigeminy
Irregularly irregular	–	Atrial fibrillation, frequent ventricular ectopics
Slow rising	Low gradient upstroke	Aortic stenosis
Waterhammer, collapsing	Steep up and down stroke (lift arm so that wrist is above heart height)	Aortic regurgitation, patent ductus arteriosus
Bisferiens	A double-peaked pulse – the second peak can be smaller, larger, or the same size as the first	Aortic regurgitation, hypertrophic cardiomyopathy
Pulsus paradoxus	An exaggerated fall in pulse volume on inspiration (>10 mm Hg on sphygmomanometry)	Cardiac tamponade, acute asthma
Bounding	Large volume	Anemia, hepatic failure, type 2 respiratory failure (high CO_2)
Pulsus alternans	Alternating large and small volume pulses	Bigeminy

Table 4. Abnormal pulses.

Blood pressure

This is described in Chapter 6, Hypertension.

Jugular venous pressure

Of all the elements of clinical examination, the jugular venous pressure (JVP) is the most mysterious. It is highly esoteric, and whilst some people wax lyrical about the steepness of the "y" descent, others will feel grateful to be convinced they see it at all. Two things are very clear: (1) the JVP is a very useful clinical marker in many situations, and (2) the exact height of the JVP is a poor guide to central venous pressure. Taken together, this suggests that noting whether the JVP is "up" or "down" is good practice in every cardiac patient. In particular, it can be very useful in diagnosing right-sided heart failure and in differentiating a cardiovascular cause of acute shortness of breath (right ventricular failure, pulmonary embolism) from an intrinsic pulmonary cause (asthma, chronic obstructive pulmonary disease). For the general physician, the waveform of the JVP (see **Figure 1**) is, for most purposes, only of academic significance.

Chapter 2

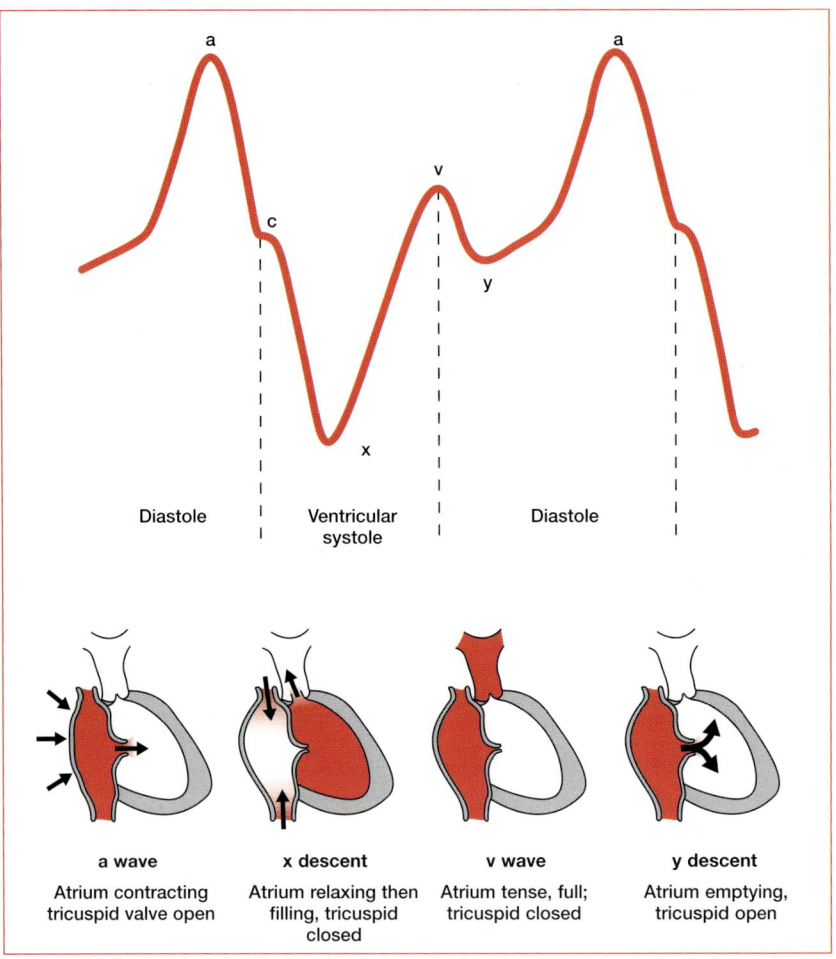

Figure 1. Waveforms of the jugular venous pressure (including a brief explanation for each wave). The "c" wave represents right ventricular contraction "pushing" the tricuspid valve back into the right atrium. Reproduced with permission from Oxford University Press (Longmore JM et al. *The Oxford Handbook of Clinical Medicine*, 5th Edn, p. 79).

The JVP should be assessed with the patient reclined at a 45° angle (see **Figure 2**). Accepted practice is that only the internal jugular vein should be used, as only this vessel joins the superior vena cava at a 180° angle. The JVP is defined as the height of the waveform in centimeters above the sternal angle (<4 cm is normal). Abnormalities of the JVP are described in **Table 5**.

Cardiovascular examination

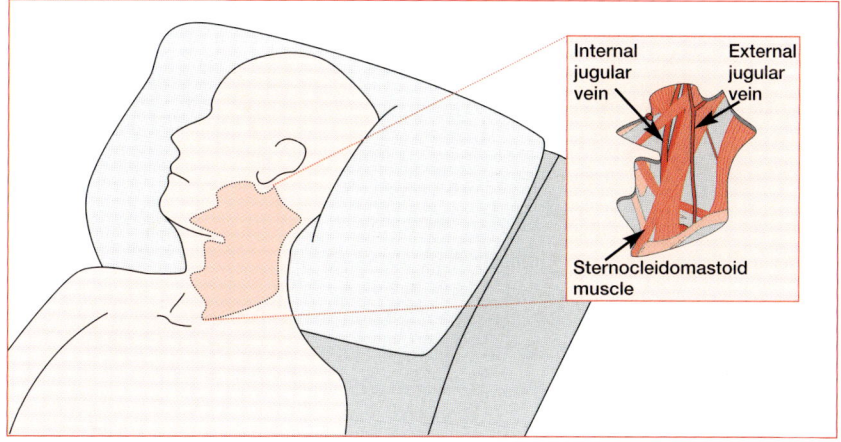

Figure 2. The jugular veins. The patient is lying at a 45° angle, thus revealing the surface markings of the neck.

JVP abnormalities	Probable cause
Large "a" wave	Tricuspid stenosis, pulmonary hypertension, pulmonary stenosis
Cannon wave	Atrial fibrillation, complete heart block, VVI pacing, ventricular tachycardia (a cannon wave occurs when the right atrium contracts against a closed tricuspid valve)
Steep "x", "y" descent	Constrictive pericarditis, cardiac tamponade
Large "v" wave, "cv" wave	Tricuspid regurgitation
Kussmaul's sign	Rise of JVP on inspiration, constrictive pericarditis, cardiac tamponade

Table 5. Abnormalities of the jugular venous pressure (JVP).

Palpation

Before auscultation, inspection of the precordium can be a useful indicator of previous surgery – eg, midline sternotomy suggests previous bypass, lateral thoracotomy suggests previous mitral valve or minimally invasive bypass surgery (left internal mammary artery to left anterior descending coronary artery). Locate the apex beat – the furthest point laterally and inferioraly where you can clearly feel the apex (usually the fifth intercostal space in the midclavicular line). There are many different descriptions for abnormal apex beats. One scheme distinguishes heaving (high afterload, eg, aortic stenosis) from thrusting (high preload, eg, aortic regurgitation). The apex may also be "tapping", but this reflects a loud first heart sound. In addition, you should place your left hand over the sternum and feel for any significant ventricular heave (right ventricular hypertrophy) or thrill (tight aortic stenosis, ventricular septal defect).

Auscultation

Held by many as the key to physical examination, the importance of auscultation remains, but is diminished in an age of increasingly portable echocardiography.

Listen over the aortic (second right intercostal space) and pulmonary (second left intercostal space) areas and at the left lower sternal edge with the diaphragm of your stethoscope (better for higher pitches), then use the bell for the apex (better for lower pitches). If in doubt, use both. Press lightly with the bell. If you hear an abnormality over the aortic or pulmonary areas, you should listen over the carotids. If you hear an abnormality at the apex, listen in the axilla. Listen systematically. Start with the heart sounds – ignore everything else.

Heart sound variations

When listening to heart sounds, note their volume (normal, diminished, loud) and whether physiological splitting is present (see **Figure 3**).

Physiological splitting of the second heart sound is when the sound of aortic valve closure (A2) occurs earlier than that of pulmonary valve closure (P2). It occurs in inspiration and is more common in the young. It is caused by increased venous return and negative intrathoracic pressure. This delays right ventricular emptying and pulmonary valve closure, at the same time that pooling of blood in the pulmonary capillary bed hastens left ventricular emptying and aortic valve closure. Reverse splitting of the second heart sound can occur in conditions where aortic valve closure is delayed, such as left bundle branch block or paced right ventricle, or where pulmonary valve closure occurs early, such as in the B form of Wolff–Parkinson–White syndrome. Wide fixed splitting of the second heart sound occurs in atrial septal defect.

A third heart sound may be heard soon after the second heart sound. It is thought to be due to rapid, high-volume filling of the left ventricle. As such, it is found in pathological (left ventricular failure) as well as physiological (athletic heart, pregnancy) states.

A fourth heart sound may be heard just before the first sound. This is caused by atrial contraction filling a stiff left ventricle, eg, hypertensive heart or diastolic heart failure.

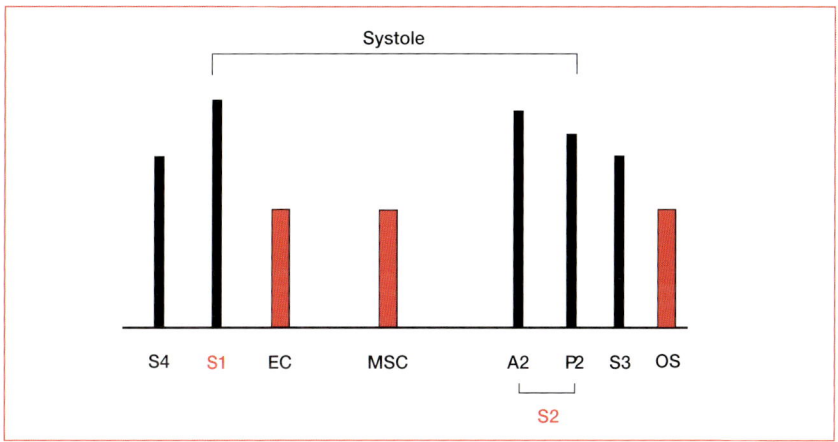

Figure 3. Relative positions of heart sounds and added sounds in auscultation. Sounds in red are high pitched. A2: aortic component of second heart sound; EC: ejection click; MSC: mid systolic click; OS: opening snap; P2: pulmonary component of second heart sound; S1–S4: heart sounds 1–4.

Murmurs

When you have considered these heart sound variations, move on to consider the gaps between the heart sounds. If you hear a murmur, first establish whether it occurs in systole or diastole (time against the carotid pulse if necessary). Then determine its length and, if short, its exact position (early, mid, or late; systole or diastole) (see **Figure 3**).

Added sounds

An opening snap occurring after the second heart sound represents a diseased mitral valve opening to a stenotic position. An ejection click soon after the first heart sound occurs in aortic stenosis and pulmonary stenosis. A mid systolic click is heard in mitral valve prolapse.

After listening to the heart

Listen to the base of the lungs for the fine inspiratory crackles of pulmonary edema. If you suspect right-sided cardiac pathology, palpate the liver, which will be enlarged, congested, and possibly pulsatile in cases of right ventricular failure or tricuspid valve disease. Also, check the patient's ankles for swelling.

Table 6 outlines common associations in cardiovascular clinical examination.

	AS	Aortic sclerosis/ minimal AS	Aortic regurgitation	Mitral stenosis	Mitral regurgitation	Tricuspid regurgitation	Pulmonary regurgitation
Pulse	Low volume, slow rising	Normal	↑ volume, collapsing	Low volume, normal/AF	Normal/AF	Normal/AF	Normal
Pulse pressure	↓	–	↑	–	–	–	–
JVP	–	–	–	–	–	↑, prominent systolic wave ("cv" wave)	–
Apex	Heaving, not displaced	Just palpable, not displaced	Thrusting, displaced	Tapping, not displaced	Thrusting, displaced	–	–
First sound	–	–	–	Loud	Soft	–	–
Second sound	Soft A2	A2 not soft	–	–	–	–	–
Added sounds	Ejection click can occur with bicuspid valve	–	–	No third sound opening snap	Third sound	–	–
Murmur	Loud, harsh, mid-systolic ejection	Ejection systolic neither harsh nor loud	Blowing, high-pitched early diastolic	Low, rumbling, mid-diastolic	Pansystolic	Pansystolic	Early diastolic
Heard best	Second right ICS	Second right ICS	LLSE (patient forward in expiration)	Apex with patient turned to left	Apex	LLSE in inspiration	Second left ICS
Radiates	Into carotids	Faintly to carotids	–	–	To axilla	–	–

Table 6. Common associations in cardiovascular clinical examination. AF: atrial fibrillation; AS: aortic stenosis; ASD: atrial septal defect; ICS: intercostal space; JVP: jugular venous pressure; LLSE: left lower sternal edge; PDA: patent ductus arteriosus; PR: pulmonary regurgitation; VSD: ventricular septal defect. See Chapter 9, Valve disease, for more on columns 1–9 and Chapter 14, Adult congenital heart disease, for columns 10–13.

Cardiovascular examination

	Tricuspid stenosis	Pulmonary stenosis	ASD	VSD	PDA	Pulmonary hypertension
Pulse	Usually low volume, AF	Low volume	Normal/AF	Normal	Regular, collapsing	Low volume, AF
Pulse pressure	–	–	–	–	↑	–
JVP	Prominent "a" wave (if sinus rhythm)	Large "a" wave	–	–	–	↑ (tricuspid regurgitation) with prominent "a" wave (if sinus rhythm)
Apex	–	–	Just palpable, not displaced	May be displaced	Thrusting, displaced	–
First sound	–	–	–	–	–	–
Second sound	–	Soft P2	Wide fixed splitting of S2	P2 may be loud	–	Loud P2
Added sounds	–	–	–	–	–	–
Murmur	Rumbling mid-diastolic	Harsh mid-systolic ejection	Ejection systolic (↑ flow across pulmonary valve) ± harsh, explosive, brief early diastolic (PR) and ejection click	Pan-systolic ± early diastolic (PR)	Continuous machinery murmur with systolic accentuation	–
Heard best	LLSE (louder on inspiration)	Second left ICS (louder on inspiration)	–	LLSE ± second left ICS	5–7 cm above and left of 2nd left ICS beneath clavicle	–
Radiates	–	–	–	Apex	Posteriorly	–

Table 6. *Continued.*

Summary

A careful clinical examination can reveal much about the condition of your patient's heart. In addition, noting the findings of a full examination will greatly facilitate specialist referral. In an age of high technology, skilled clinical examination has yet to be surpassed in terms of convenience, safety, and value for money.

Further reading

Bickley LS, Hoekelman RA, editors. *Bates' Pocket Guide to Physical Examination and History Taking*, 3rd edn. Lippincott Williams & Wilkins, 2000.

Gleadle J. *History and Examination at a Glance*. Blackwell Science, 2003

Perloff JK. *Physical Examination of the Heart and Circulation*, 3rd edn. WB Saunders, 2000.

Turner RC, Blackwood RA. *Lecture Notes on Clinical Skills*, 3rd edn. Blackwell Science, 1997.

Chapter 3

Conquering the ECG

Besides the stethoscope, the electrocardiogram (ECG) is the oldest and most enduring tool of the cardiologist. A basic knowledge of the ECG will enhance the understanding of cardiology (not to mention this book).

Electrocardiography

At every beat, the heart is depolarized to trigger its contraction. This electrical activity is transmitted throughout the body and can be picked up on the skin. This is the principle behind the ECG. An ECG machine records this activity via electrodes on the skin and displays it graphically. An ECG involves attaching 10 electrical cables to the body: one to each limb and six across the chest.

ECG terminology has two meanings for the word "lead":

- the cable used to connect an electrode to the ECG recorder
- the electrical view of the heart obtained from any one combination of electrodes

---

Carrying out an ECG

1) Ask the patient to undress down to the waist and lie down
2) Remove excess hair where necessary
3) Attach limb leads (anywhere on the limb)
4) Attach the chest leads (see **Figure 1**) as follows:

- V1 and V2: either side of the sternum on the fourth rib (count down from the sternal angle, the second rib insertion)
- V4: on the apex of the heart (feel for it)
- V3: halfway between V2 and V4
- V5 and V6: horizontally laterally from V4 (not up towards the axilla)

5) Ask the patient to relax
6) Press record

15

Chapter 3

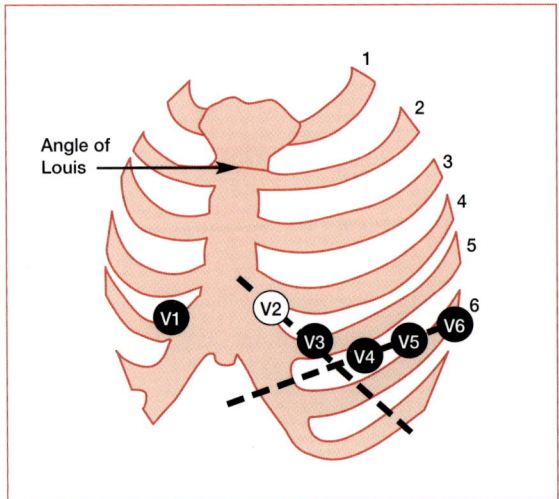

Figure 1. Standard attachment sites for chest leads.

The standard ECG uses 10 cables to obtain 12 electrical views of the heart. The different views reflect the angles at which electrodes "look" at the heart and the direction of the heart's electrical depolarization.

Limb leads

Three bipolar leads and three unipolar leads are obtained from three electrodes attached to the left arm, the right arm, and the left leg, respectively. (An electrode is also attached to the right leg, but this is an earth electrode.) The bipolar limb leads reflect the potential difference between two of the three limb electrodes:

- **lead I**: right arm–left arm
- **lead II**: right arm–left leg
- **lead III**: left leg–left arm

The unipolar leads reflect the potential difference between one of the three limb electrodes and an estimate of zero potential – derived from the remaining two limb electrodes. These leads are known as augmented leads. The augmented leads and their respective limb electrodes are:

- **aVR lead**: right arm
- **aVL lead**: left arm
- **aVF lead**: left leg

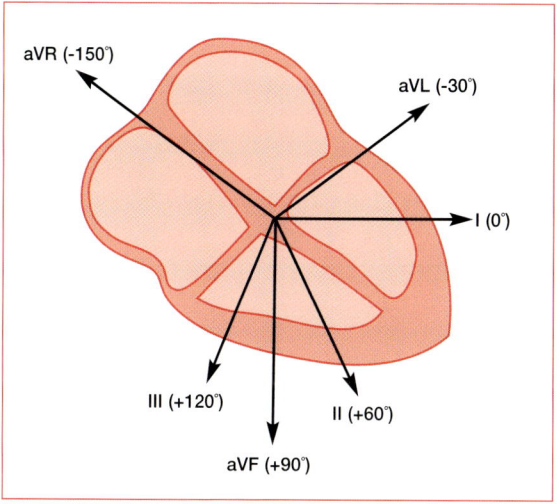

Figure 2. The limb leads looking at the heart in a vertical plane.

View	Lead
Inferior	II, III, aVF
Anterior	I, aVL, V1–V3
Septal	V3, V4
Lateral	V4–V6

Table 1. ECG leads and their respective views of the heart.

Chest leads

Another six electrodes, placed in standard positions on the chest wall, give rise to a further six unipolar leads – the chest leads (also known as precordial leads), V1–V6. The potential difference of a chest lead is recorded between the relevant chest electrode and an estimate of zero potential – derived from the average potential recorded from the three limb leads.

Planes of view

The limb leads look at the heart in a vertical plane (see **Figure 2**), whereas the chest leads look at the heart in a horizontal plane. In this way, a three-dimensional electrical picture of the heart is built up (see **Table 1**).

17

Chapter 3

> **PERFORMING DOGS**
>
> *British physiologist Augustus D Waller of St Mary's Medical School, London, published the first human electrocardiogram in the British Medical Journal in 1888. It was recorded from Thomas Goswell, a technician in the laboratory, using a capillary electrometer. After that, Waller used a more available subject for his demonstrations – his dog Jimmy, who would patiently stand with his paws in glass jars of saline.*

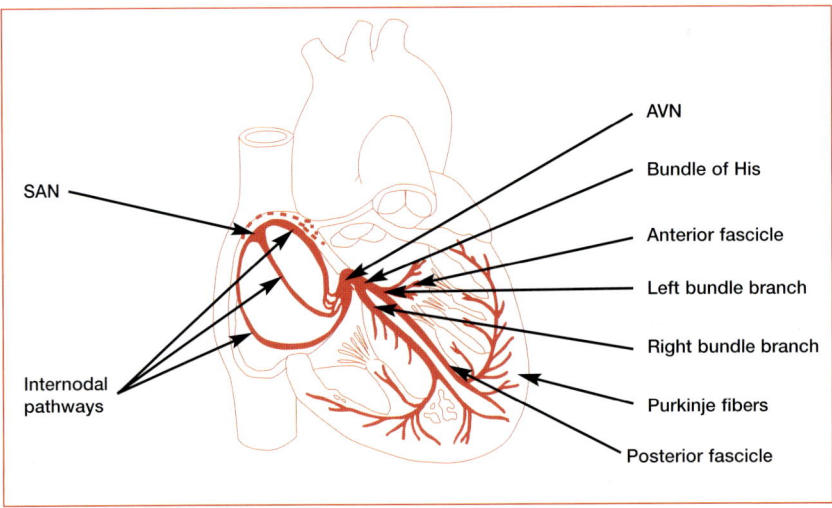

Figure 3. The cardiac depolarization route. AVN: atrioventricular node; SAN: sinoatrial node. Reproduced with permission from WB Saunders (Guyton A, Hall J. *Textbook of Medical Physiology*. Philadelphia: WB Saunders, 1996).

Depolarization of the heart

The route that the depolarization wave takes across the heart is outlined in **Figure 3**. The sinoatrial node (SAN) is the heart's pacemaker. From the SAN, the wave of depolarization spreads across the atria to the atrioventricular node (AVN). The impulse is delayed briefly at the AVN and atrial contraction is completed.

The wave of depolarization then proceeds rapidly to the bundle of His where it splits into two pathways and travels along the right and left bundle branches. The impulse travels the length of the bundles along the interventricular septum to the base of the heart, where the bundles divide into the Purkinje system. From here, the wave of depolarization is distributed to the ventricular walls and initiates ventricular contraction.

Conquering the ECG

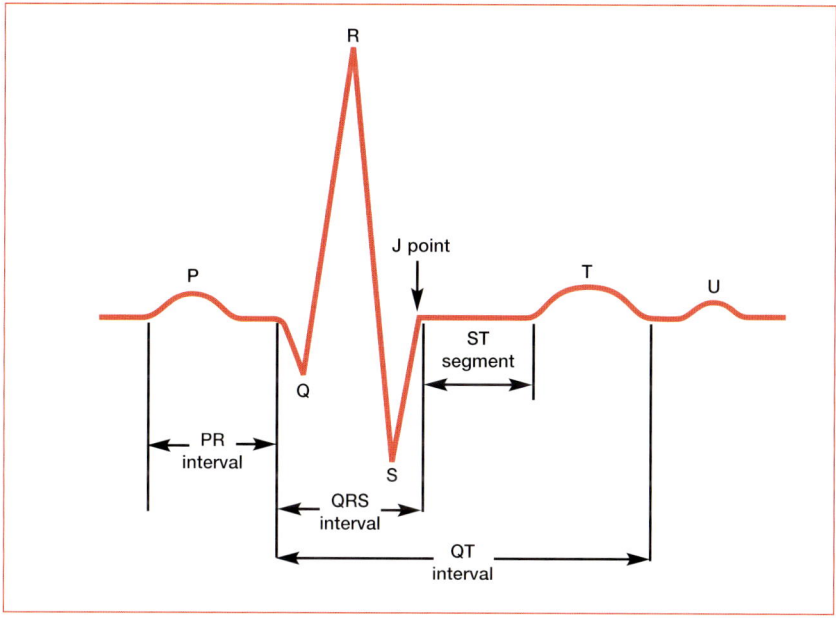

Figure 4. The basic pattern of electrical activity across the heart.

The ECG trace

The ECG machine processes the signals picked up from the skin by electrodes and produces a graphic representation of the electrical activity of the patient's heart. The basic pattern of the ECG is logical:

- electrical activity towards a lead causes an upward deflection
- electrical activity away from a lead causes a downward deflection
- depolarization and repolarization deflections occur in opposite directions

The basic pattern of this electrical activity was first discovered over a hundred years ago. It comprises three waves, which have been named P, QRS (a wave complex), and T (see **Figure 4**).

P wave
The P wave is a small deflection wave that represents atrial depolarization.

PR interval
The PR interval is the time between the first deflection of the P wave and the first deflection of the QRS complex.

19

Chapter 3

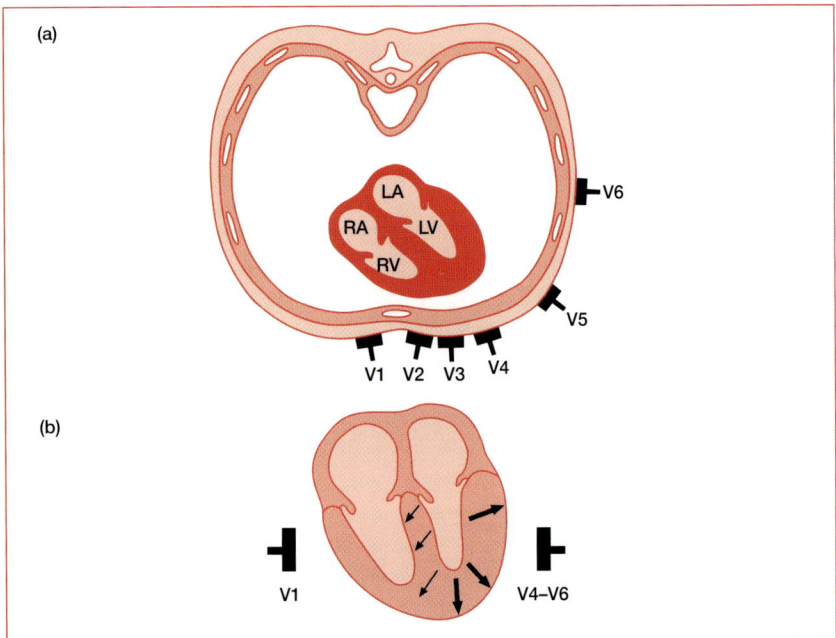

Figure 5. (a) A horizontal section through the chest showing the orientation of the chest leads with respect to the chambers of the heart. (b) In lead V1, depolarization of the interventricular septum occurs towards the lead, thus creating an upward deflection (R wave) on the ECG. It is followed by depolarization of the main mass of the LV, which occurs away from the lead, thus creating a downward deflection (S wave). This pattern is reversed for lead V6, explaining the different shapes of the QRS complex. This pattern should be checked in every ECG. LA: left atrium; LV: left ventricle; RA: right atrium; RV: right ventricle.

QRS wave complex

The three waves of the QRS complex represent ventricular depolarization. For the inexperienced, one of the most confusing aspects of ECG reading is the labeling of these waves. The rule is: if the wave immediately after the P wave is an upward deflection, it is an R wave; if it is a downward deflection, it is a Q wave:

- small Q waves correspond to depolarization of the interventricular septum. Q waves can also relate to breathing and are generally small and thin. They can also signal an old myocardial infarction (in which case they are big and wide)
- the R wave reflects depolarization of the main mass of the ventricles – hence it is the largest wave
- the S wave signifies the final depolarization of the ventricles, at the base of the heart

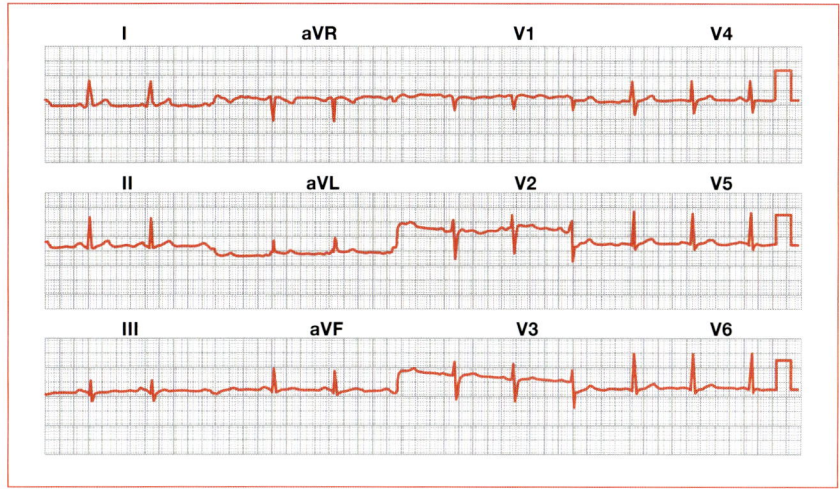

Figure 6. Example of a normal ECG.

ST segment
The ST segment, which is also known as the ST interval, is the time between the end of the QRS complex and the start of the T wave. It reflects the period of zero potential between ventricular depolarization and repolarization.

T wave
T waves represent ventricular repolarization (atrial repolarization is obscured by the large QRS complex).

Wave direction and size
Since the direction of a deflection, upward or downward, is dependent on whether the electrical activity is going towards or away from a lead, it differs according to the orientation of the lead with respect to the heart (see **Figure 5**).

The ECG trace reflects the net electrical activity at a given moment. Consequently, activity in one direction is masked if there is more activity, eg, by a larger mass, in the other direction. For example, the left ventricle muscle mass is much greater than the right, and therefore its depolarization accounts for the direction of the biggest wave.

Interpreting the ECG
A normal ECG tracing is provided in **Figure 6**. The only way to become confident at reading ECGs is to practice. It is important to be methodical – every ECG reading should start with an assessment of the rate, rhythm, and axis. This approach always reveals something about an ECG, regardless of how unusual it is.

Chapter 3

Number of large squares between QRS complexes	Heart rate (bpm)
5	60
4	75
3	100
2	150

Table 2. Some common heart rates as determined by analysis of the QRS complex.

Rate
Identify the QRS complex (this is generally the biggest wave); count the number of large squares between one QRS wave and the next; divide 300 by this number to determine the rate (see **Table 2**).

Rhythm
P waves are the key to determining whether a patient is in sinus rhythm or not. If P waves are not clearly visible in the chest leads, look for them in the other leads. The presence of P waves immediately before every QRS complex indicates sinus rhythm. If there are no P waves, note whether the QRS complexes are wide or narrow, regular or irregular.

No P waves and irregular narrow QRS complexes
This is the hallmark of atrial fibrillation (see **Figure 7**). Sometimes the baseline appears "noisy" and sometimes it appears entirely flat. However, if there are no P waves and the QRS complexes appear at randomly irregular intervals, the diagnosis is atrial fibrillation.

Sawtooth P waves
A sawtooth waveform signifies atrial flutter (see **Figure 8**). The number of atrial contractions to one ventricular contraction should be specified.

Axis
The axis is the net direction of electrical activity during depolarization. It is altered by left ventricular or right ventricular hypertrophy or by bundle branch blocks. It is a very straightforward measurement that, once it has been grasped, can be calculated instantaneously:

- find the QRS complex in the I and aVF leads (because these look at the heart at 0° and +90°, respectively)
- determine the net positivity of the QRS wave from each of the two leads by subtracting the S wave height (the number of small squares that it crosses

Conquering the ECG

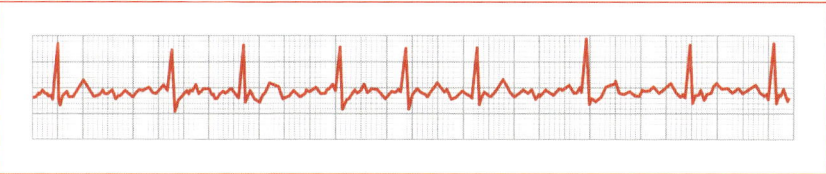

Figure 7. ECG demonstrating atrial fibrillation.

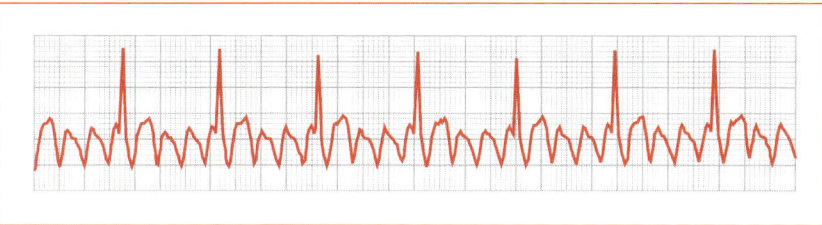

Figure 8. ECG demonstrating atrial flutter – note the characteristic sawtooth waveform.

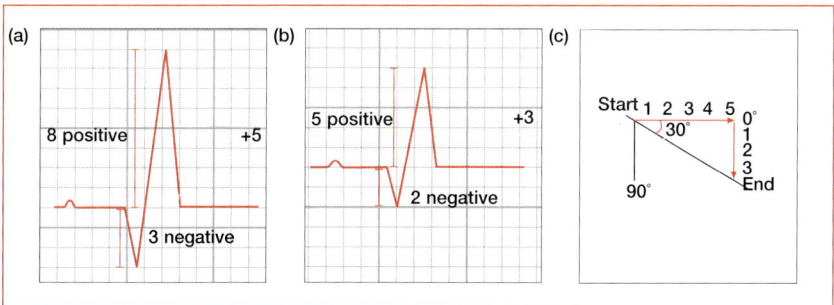

Figure 9. Vector diagram to determine the QRS axis.

as it dips below the baseline – if it does) from the R wave height (the number of small squares that it crosses as it rises) (see **Figure 9a** and **9b**)
- plot out the net sizes of these QRS waves against each other on a vector diagram (see **Figure 9c**). For the I lead, plot net positives to the right and net negatives to the left; for the aVF lead, plot positive downwards and negative upwards
- the direction of the endpoint from the starting point represents the axis or predominant direction of electrical depolarization (determined primarily by the muscle mass of the left ventricle). It is expressed as an angle and can be estimated quite easily (normal is 0°–120°)

23

Chapter 3

> **HUMAN RESUSCITATION**
>
> The first electrical resuscitation of a human took place (almost certainly) in 1872. The resuscitation of a drowned girl with electricity is described by Guillaume Benjamin Amand Duchenne de Boulogne, a pioneering neurophysiologist, in the third edition of his textbook on the medical uses of electricity. Although it is sometimes described as the first artificial pacing, the stimulation was of the phrenic nerve and not the myocardium.

ECG abnormalities

This section discusses the most important and most frequently encountered ECG abnormalities.

Normal variations

- Small Q waves and inverted T waves in lead III often disappear on deep inspiration. Occasional septal Q waves can be seen in other leads.
- ST elevation following an S wave ("high take off") is common in leads V2–V4 and is quite normal. Differentiating this from pathological ST elevation can be difficult and relies on the patient's history and the availability of a previous ECG. These "repolarization abnormalities" are more common in the young and in athletes.
- T-wave inversion is common in Afro-Caribbean blacks.
- U waves – small extra waves following T waves – are seen in hypokalemic patients, but can also represent a normal variant.
- Ventricular extrasystoles – no P waves, broad and abnormal QRS complexes, and T waves interspersed between normal sinus rhythm – sometimes occur and do not require further investigation unless they are associated with symptoms (such as dizziness, palpitations, exercise intolerance, chest pain, shortness of breath) or occur several times every minute.

Pathological variations

Long PR interval

A distance of more than five small squares from the start of the P wave to the start of the R wave (or Q wave if there is one) constitutes first-degree heart block (see **Figure 10**). It rarely requires action, but in the presence of other abnormalities might be a sign of hyperkalemia, digoxin toxicity, or cardiomyopathy.

Conquering the ECG

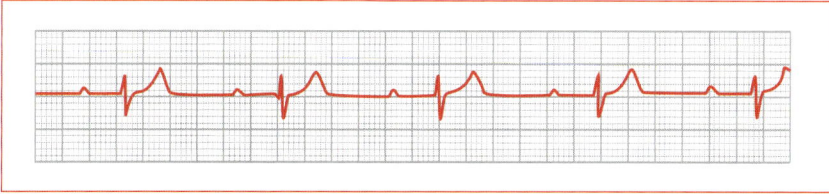

Figure 10. ECG demonstrating first-degree heart block.

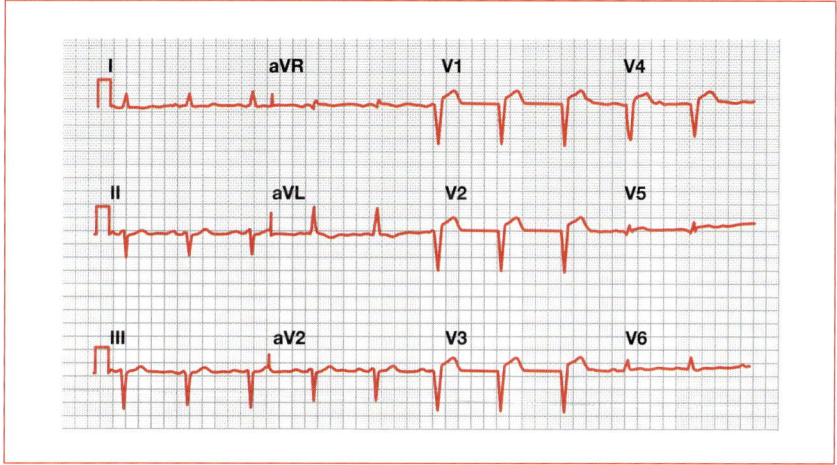

Figure 11. ECG demonstrating abnormal Q waves in V1–V4. This is indicative of a previous infarction.

EKG OR ECG?

There is some debate over exactly who invented the electrocardiogram. The Dutch "K" (elektrokardiogram) is often used as a tribute to the Indonesian-born physician Wilhelm Einthoven who, while working in The Netherlands in 1924, received the Nobel prize for "the discovery of the mechanism of the electrocardiogram". In fact, it was Augustus Désiré Waller, a physician trained in Edinburgh, who presented – to the students of St Mary's Hospital medical school, London, at the introductory lecture of the 1888 academic year – his "cardiograph", the first ever ECG recording in man. It was some years later, in 1901, that Wilhelm Einthoven reported his string galvanometer – with the limb leads labeled I, II, and III and the waves labeled P, QRS, and T as we know them today. In fact, although often credited with inventing the term electrocardiogram (which is why it is sometimes spelt the Dutch way), Einthoven credits Waller with this distinction in his 1895 publication in Pflügers Archives "Über die Form des menschlichen Elektrokardiogramms".

Chapter 3

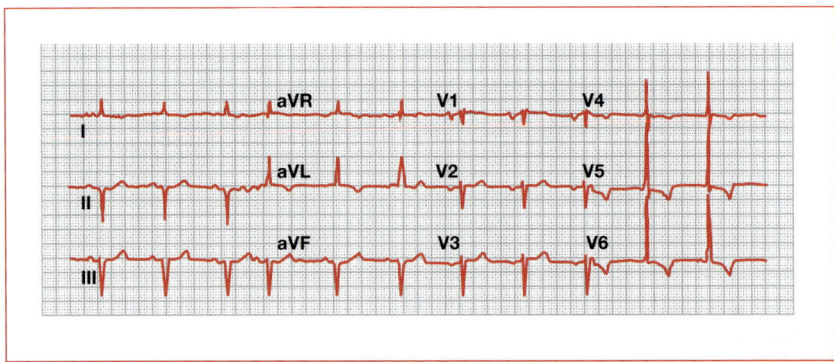

Figure 12. ECG demonstrating left ventricular hypertrophy. Note also the T-wave inversion in leads V4–V6. This is often labeled "strain".

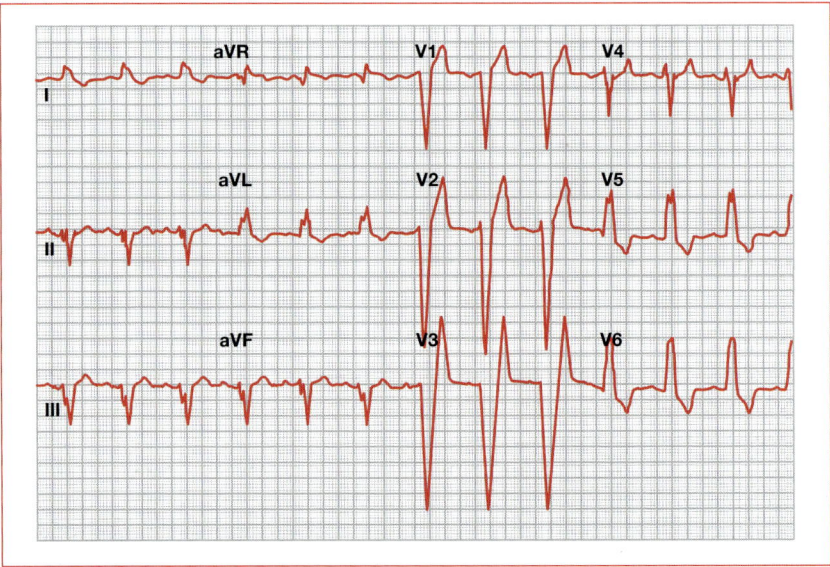

Figure 13. ECG demonstrating left bundle branch block.

Q waves

A normal ECG has only very small Q waves. A downward deflection immediately following a P wave that is wider than two small squares or greater in height than a third of the subsequent R wave is significant: such Q waves can represent previous infarction (see **Figure 11**, previous page).

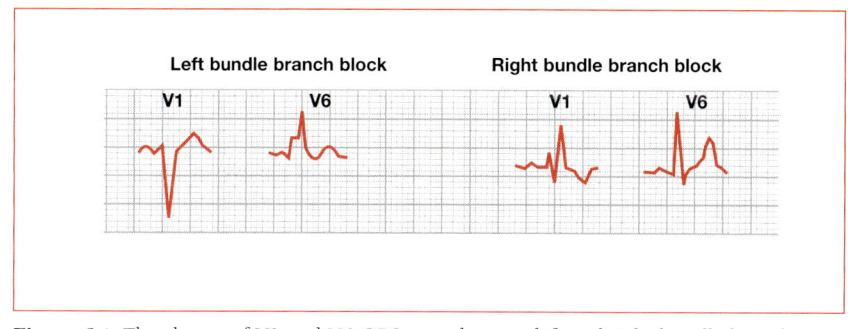

Figure 14. The shapes of V1 and V6 QRS complexes in left and right bundle branch block.

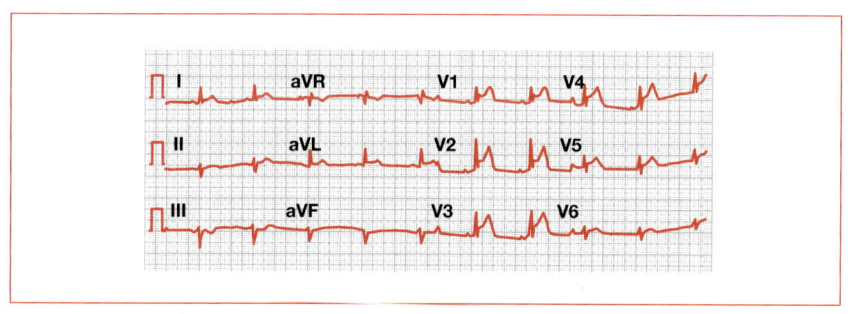

Figure 15. ECG demonstrating anteroseptal myocardial infarction. Note the ST-segment elevation.

Large QRS complexes

Left ventricular hypertrophy (LVH) is one of the easiest and most useful diagnoses to make (see **Figure 12**). The Sokolow–Lyon index is the most commonly calculated index of estimation. Does the sum of the S wave in lead V1 (SV1) and the R wave in V6 (RV6) add up to more than 3.5 mV, ie, 35 small or seven big squares? If so, the patient has LVH by voltage criterion. Right ventricular hypertrophy is indicated by a dominant R wave in V1 (ie, R wave bigger than following S wave; Sokolow–Lyon index: R in V1 + S in V5 or V6 ≥ 1.05 mV) and right axis deviation.

Broad QRS complexes and strange-looking ECGs

A wide QRS complex despite sinus rhythm is the hallmark of bundle branch block. Left bundle branch block (LBBB) can cause the ECG to look extremely abnormal (see **Figure 13**). When faced with such an ECG – after calculating rate, rhythm, and axis – check the width of the QRS complex. If it is more than three small squares wide, it is abnormal. Bundle branch block can then be diagnosed by pattern recognition of the QRS complexes in the V1 and V6 leads (see **Figure 14**). New LBBB can be diagnostic of myocardial infarction (MI).

Chapter 3

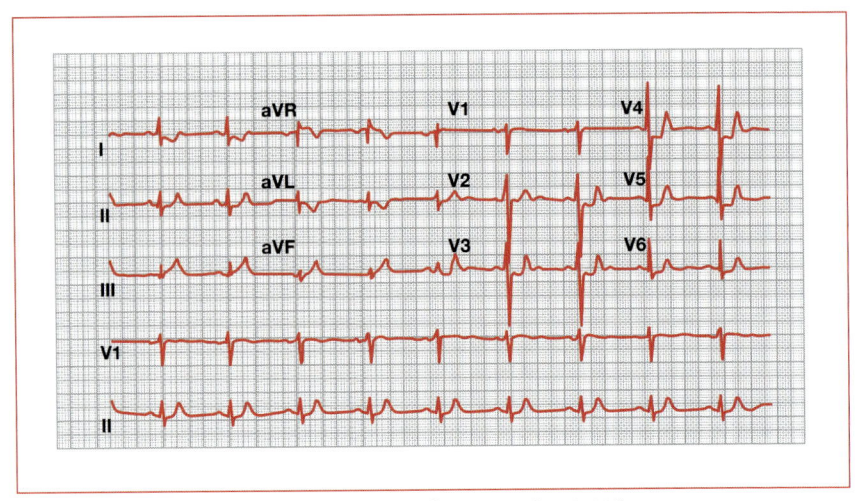

Figure 16. ECG demonstrating ST-segment depression (I, V3–V6).

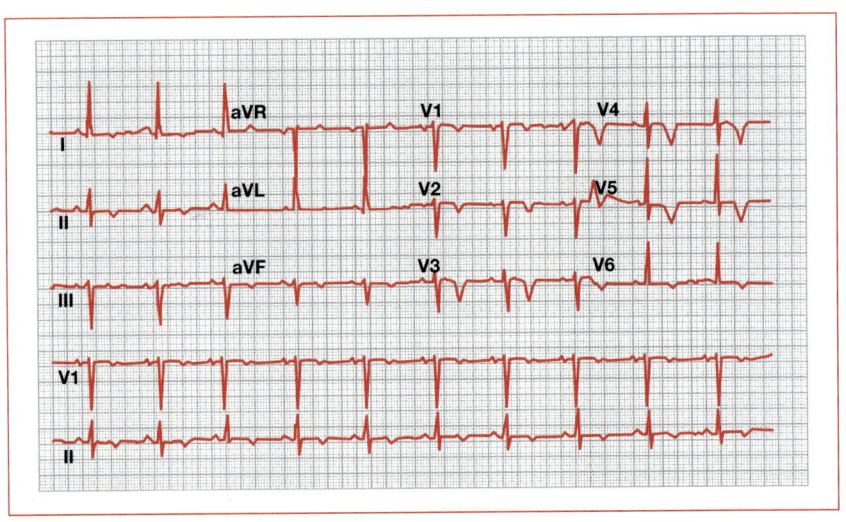

Figure 17. ECG demonstrating T-wave inversion.

ST segment changes

The ST segment extends from the end of the S wave to the start of the T wave. It should be flat or slightly upsloping and level with the baseline. Elevation of more than two small squares in the chest leads or one small square in the limb leads, combined with a characteristic history, indicates the possibility of MI (see **Figure 15**, previous page). ST depression is diagnostic of ischemia (see **Figure 16**). It is worth noting that although ST elevation can localize the lesion (eg, anterior MI,

Conquering the ECG

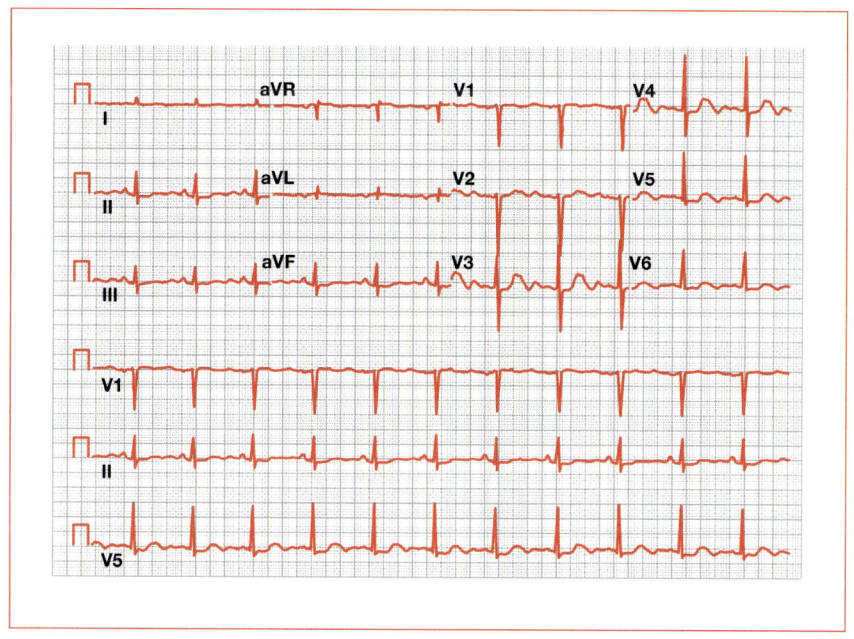

Figure 18. ECG demonstrating a long QT interval.

inferior MI), ST depression cannot. Concave upwards ST elevation in all 12 leads is diagnostic of pericarditis.

T waves
In a normal ECG, T waves are upright in every lead except aVR. T-wave inversion can represent current ischemia or previous infarction (see **Figure 17**). In combination with LVH and ST depression, it can represent "strain". This form of LVH carries a poor prognosis.

Long QT interval
The QT interval should be less than half of the R–R interval. Calculation of the corrected QT (QTc) is generally not necessary and usually will have been done by the ECG machine (but beware of blindly believing any automated diagnostic system). Conditions associated with a long QT interval are outlined in **Table 3** (see **Figure 18**).

Long QT syndrome may also be drug-induced (see **Table 4**, p. 32). Once this occurs, the responsible drug needs to be discontinued.

Chapter 3

Congenital	Acquired
Jervell and Lange–Nielsen syndrome	Amiodarone, sotalol
Romano–Ward syndrome	Flecainide
	Hypocalcemia
	Hypokalemia
	Hypomagnesemia
	Phenothiazines
	Tricyclic antidepressants

Table 3. Causes of a long QT interval.

Pattern combinations
Digoxin
A reverse tick ST depression is characteristic and does not indicate toxicity. Digoxin toxicity can result in dysrhythmia.

Pulmonary embolism
Sinus tachycardia is seen in many patients with pulmonary embolism. New right bundle branch block (RBBB) or right axis deviation with "strain" can also indicate PE. The classic $S_I Q_{III} T_{III}$ is less common.

Hyperkalemia
The absolute potassium level is less important than its rate of rise. ECG changes reflecting a rapid rise demand immediate action (see **Figures 19–21**). The level of danger increases as the ECG changes progress. The sequence generally follows the order:

- tall, tented T waves (see **Figure 19**)
- lengthening of the PR interval
- reduction in the P-wave height
- widening of the QRS complex (see **Figure 20**)
- "sinus" wave QRS pattern (see **Figure 21**)

A sinus-wave QRS should be treated immediately with calcium chloride, whilst hyperkalemia associated with lesser ECG changes can be treated with insulin/glucose infusion.

Conquering the ECG

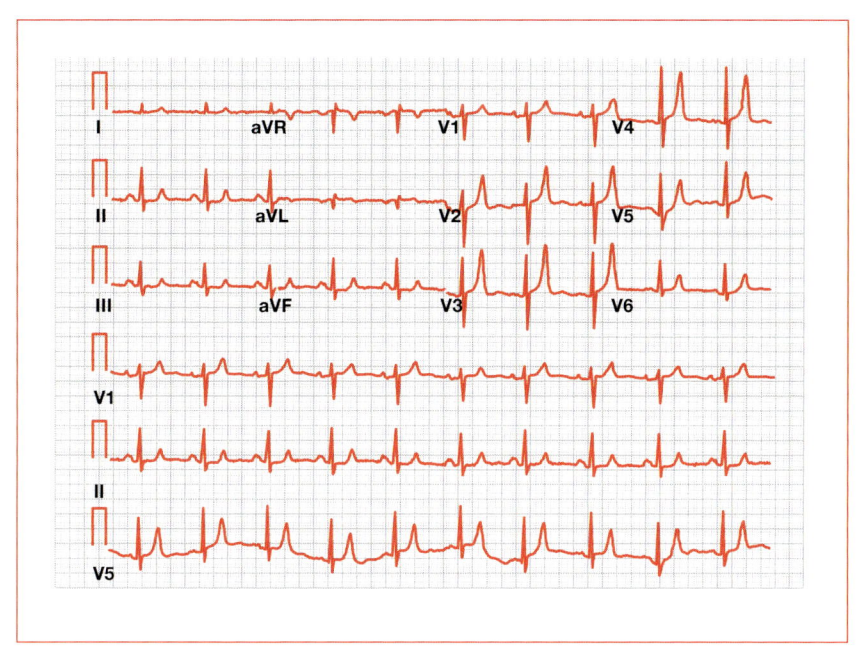

Figure 19. Hyperkalemia. Note the tall, tented T waves.

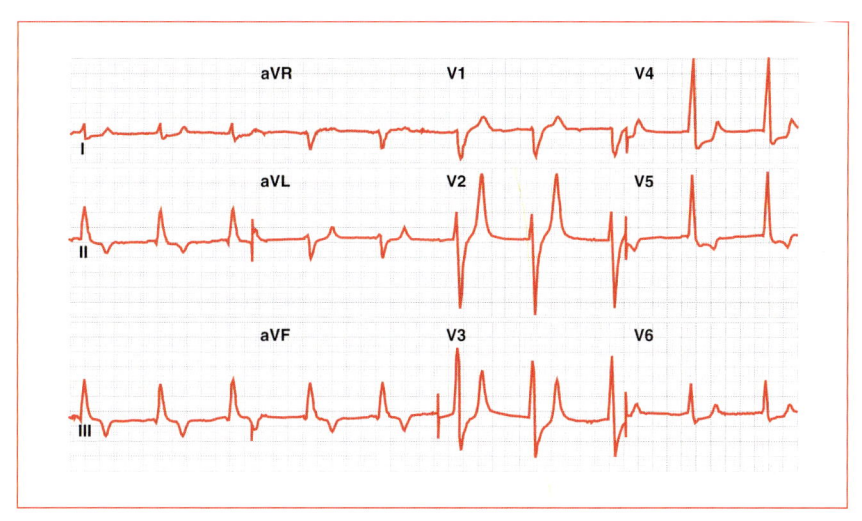

Figure 20. ECG demonstrating a widening of the QRS complex.

Chapter 3

Generic name	QT interval	Torsade de pointes	Generic name	QT interval	Torsade de pointes
Antiarrhythmics			**Selective serotonin re-uptake inhibitors**		
Ajmaline	+	+	Fluoxetine	+	+
Amiodarone	+	+	Paroxetine	+	
Chinidine	+	+	Sertraline	+	+
Disopyramide	+	+	**Anticonvulsants**		
Dofetilide	+	+	Valproate	+	
Ibutilide	+	+	**Other psychopharmaceuticals**		
Propafenone	+	+	Chloralhydrate	+	+
Sotalol	+	+	Levomethadone	+	+
Antibiotics (macrolides)			Lithium	+	
Azithromycin		+	Naratriptan	+	
Clarithromycin	+	+	Sumatriptan	+	
Clindamycin		+	Venlafaxine	+	
Erythromycin	+	+	Zolmitriptan	+	
Roxithromycin	+		**Anti-Parkinson's**		
Spiramycin	+	+	Amantadine		+
Antibiotics (quinolones)			Budipine[c]	+	+
Gatifloxacin	+	+	**Antimalarials**		
Grepafloxacin[a]	+	+	Quinine	+	+
Levofloxacin		+	Chloroquine	+	+
Moxifloxacin	+	+	Halofantrine	+	
Sparfloxacin	+	+	Mefloquine	+	
Other antibiotics			**Diuretics**		
Amoxicillin	+		Indapamide	+	
Trimethoprim-sulfamethoxazole		+	**Lipid-lowering agents**		
Antihistamines			Probucol	+	+
Astemizole[a]	+	+	**Motility enhancers**		
Clemastine	+		Cisapride[a]	+	+
Diphenhydramine	+		**Nootropic geriatrics**		
Hydroxyzine	+		Vincamine	+	
Terfenadine	+	+	**Chemotherapeutics**		
Antidepressants			Tamoxifen	+	+
Amitriptyline	+	+	Pentamidine	+	+
Clomipramine	+		**Immunosuppressants**		
Desipramine	+	+	Tacrolimus	+	+
Doxepine	+		**Peptides**		
Imipramine	+	+	Octreotide	+	
Maprotiline	+	+	**Virostatics**		
Neuroleptics			Foscarnet	+	
Amisulpride	+		**Muscle relaxants**		
Clozapine	+		Tizanidine	+	
Chlorpromazine	+	+	**X-ray contrast agents**		
Droperidol[a]	+	+	Ioxaglate meglumine	+	+
Fluphenazine	+				
Haloperidol	+	+			
Melperone	+	+			
Olanzapine	+				
Pimozide	+	+			
Quetiapine	+				
Sulpiride	+	+			
Thioridazine	+	+			
Risperidone	+				
Sertindole[b]	+	+			
Tiapride	+	+			
Trazodone	+				

Table 4. Drug-induced increase in the QT interval and torsade de pointes.
+ A prolonged QT interval can occur or torsade de pointes was observed.
[a]Taken off the market.
[b]Suspended from the market, final decision by the regulatory authorities still awaited.
[c]Indication limitations have been expressed.
Important tips on the use of the table: information is based on the latest scientific knowledge as far as it is generally available from published studies (Medline research), case reports, internet publications, specialist information, the Red List, and information from the regulatory authorities. In the case reports available about torsade de pointes, the causal relationship to the ingestion of the particular medication is no longer apparent; pure coincidence cannot be excluded in individual cases.

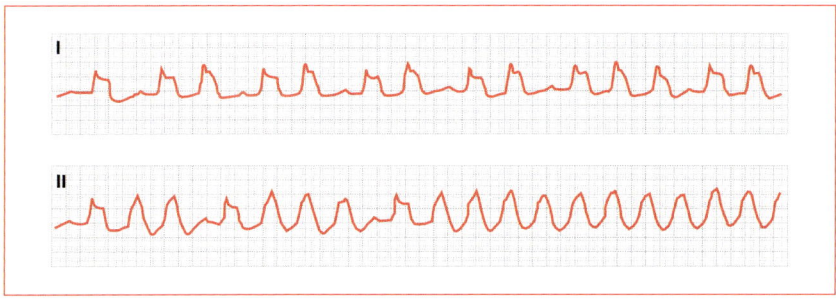

Figure 21. ECG demonstrating a sinus-wave QRS pattern.

> **PQRST?**
>
> Nobody knows for sure why these letters became standard. Certainly, mathematicians used to start lettering systems from the middle of the alphabet to avoid confusion with the frequently used letters at the beginning. Einthoven used the letters O to X to mark the timeline on his ECG diagrams and, of course, P is the letter that follows O. If the image of the PQRST diagram was striking enough to be adopted by researchers as a true representation of the underlying form, it would have been logical to continue the same naming convention when the more advanced string galvanometer started creating ECGs a few years later.

Further reading

Ashley EA, Raxwal VK, Froelicher VF. The prevalence and prognostic significance of electrocardiographic abnormalities. *Curr Probl Cardiol* 2000;25:1–72.

Hampton JR. *ECG Made Easy*. London: Churchill Livingstone, 1997.

Rautaharju PM. A hundred years of progress in electrocardiography. 1: Early contributions from Waller to Wilson. *Can J Cardiol* 1987;3:362–74.

Chapter 4

Understanding the echocardiogram

Although few generalists actually perform echocardiograms, most order or have to interpret them at some stage. Our aim then is not to explain how to carry out echocardiography, but how to realize its potential and limitations.

Background

"Ultra" sound has a frequency above the range audible by humans (ie, >20,000 Hz). For adult cardiac imaging, ultrasound waves in the range of 4–7 MHz are used (intravascular ultrasound uses frequencies as high as 30 MHz). These are created within the ultrasound probe by striking piezo-electric crystals with an electric pulse, which stimulates the crystals to release sound waves. The central principle of ultrasound imaging is that, while most waves are absorbed by the body, those at interfaces between different tissue densities are reflected. In addition to emitting the ultrasound waves, the transducer detects the returning waves, processes the information, and displays it as characteristic images. Higher frequency ultrasound waves increase resolution, but decrease tissue penetration.

Imaging modes

There are three basic "modes" used to image the heart:

- two-dimensional (2D) imaging
- M-mode imaging
- Doppler imaging

Two-dimensional imaging

2D imaging is the mainstay of echo imaging and allows structures to be viewed moving in real time in a cross-section of the heart (two dimensions). It is used for detecting abnormal anatomy or abnormal movement of structures. The most common cross-sectional views are the parasternal long axis, the parasternal short axis, and the apical view (see **Figure 1**). The gastric or subcostal and suprasternal views are also commonly used.

Chapter 4

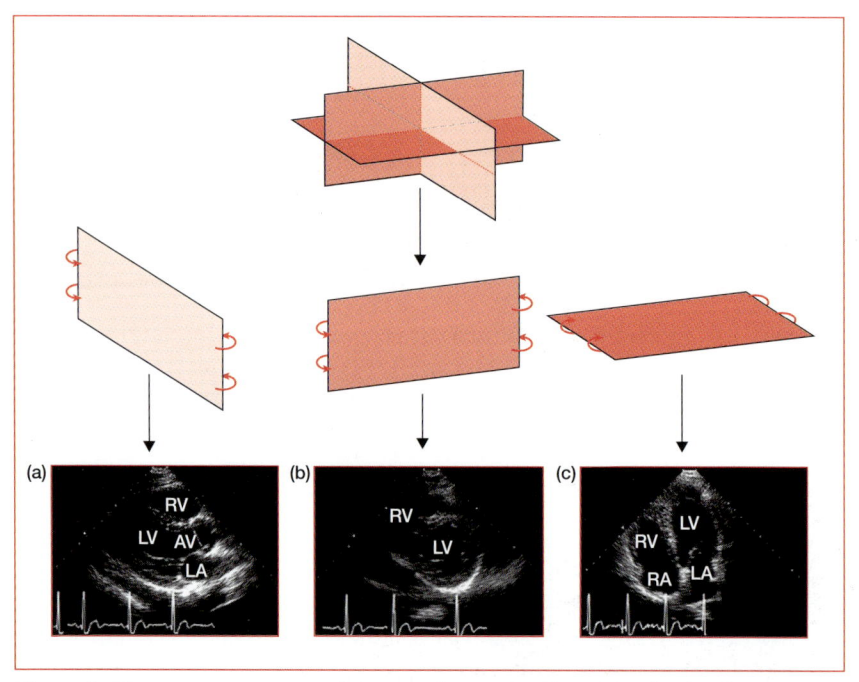

Figure 1. The most common two-dimensional imaging echo views. The first line illustrates the three planes (think of them as three plates of glass intersecting at 90°), the second line shows these three planes separated, and the third line shows the accompanying echo views. (**a**) Parasternal long axis; (**b**) parasternal short axis; (**c**) apical 4-chamber view (note, in the UK, the 4-chamber view is shown upside down). AV: aortic valve; LA: left atrium; LV: left ventricle; RA: right atrium; RV: right ventricle.

M-mode imaging

The M-mode echo, which provides a 1D view, is used for fine measurements. Temporal and spatial resolutions are higher because the focus is on only one of the lines from the 2D trace (see **Figure 2**).

Doppler imaging

The concept of Doppler imaging is familiar to all those who have heard the note of a police siren change as it moves past them – as the police siren travels towards you, the frequency of the wave (pitch) appears to be higher than if it was stationary; as the siren travels away, the pitch appears to be lower.

Estimates of blood-flow velocity can be made by comparing the frequency change between the transmitted and reflected sound waves. In cardiac ultrasound, Doppler is used in three ways:

Understanding the echocardiogram

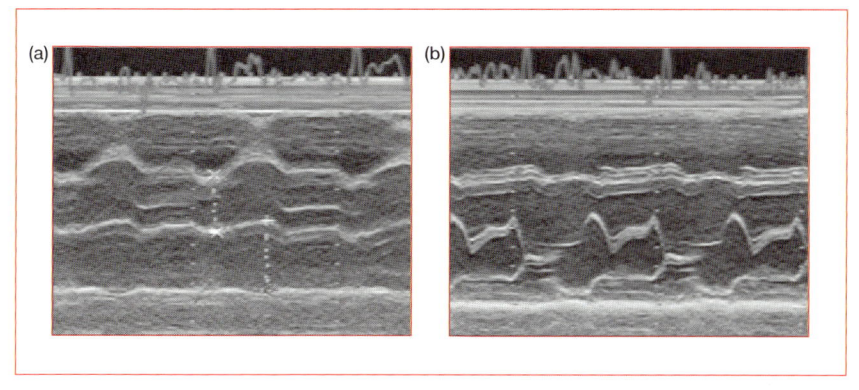

Figure 2. M-mode image of (**a**) the aorta/left atrium and (**b**) the mitral valve, both in a healthy heart.

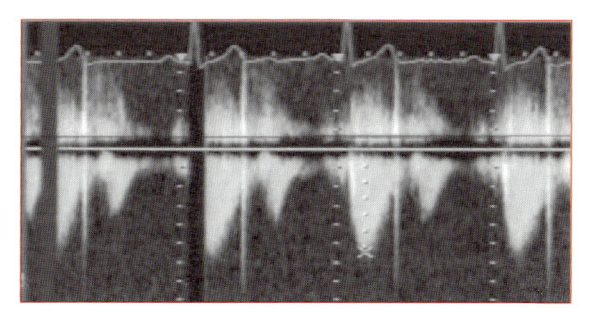

Figure 3. Continuous-wave Doppler signal.

- continuous-wave (CW) Doppler
- pulsed-wave (PW) Doppler
- color-flow mapping (CFM)

Continuous-wave Doppler
CW Doppler is sensitive, but, because it measures velocity along the entire length of the ultrasound beam and not at a specific depth, it does not localize velocity measurements of blood flow. It is used to estimate the severity of valve stenosis or regurgitation by assessing the shape or density of the output (see **Figure 3**).

Pulsed-wave Doppler
PW Doppler was developed because of the need to make localized velocity measurements of turbulent flow (it measures the blood-flow velocity within a small area at a specified tissue depth). It is used to assess ventricular in-flow patterns, intracardiac shunts, and to make precise measurements of blood flow at valve orifices.

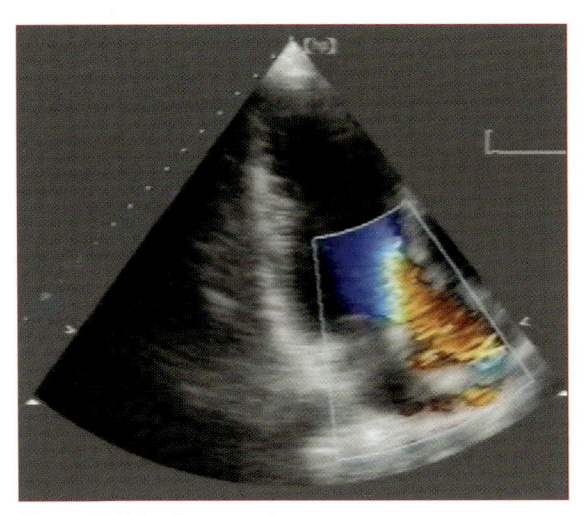

Figure 4. Color-flow mapping.

Color-flow mapping
CFM uses measurements of the velocity and direction of blood flow to superimpose a color pattern onto a section of a 2D image (see **Figure 4**). Traditionally, flow towards the transducer is red, flow away from the transducer is blue, and higher velocities are shown in lighter shades. To aid observation of turbulent flow there is a threshold velocity, above which the color changes (in some systems to green). This leads to a "mosaic" pattern at the site of turbulent flow and enables sensitive screening for regurgitant flow.

Transesophageal echocardiography

Transesophageal echocardiography (TEE) is usually carried out under mild sedation with midazolam. A thin probe is passed down the esophagus until it is level with the heart. This position provides especially clear views. It is particularly useful for imaging posterior cardiac structures. The key indications for TEE are:

- infective endocarditis – if vegetations are not seen on transthoracic echo, but suspicion is high, or with prosthetic valves
- to rule out an embolic source (especially in atrial fibrillation)
- acute dissection
- mitral valve (MV) disease preoperatively

Contrast echocardiography

Contrast echo can be useful for confirming a diagnosis of atrial septal defect (ASD). Agitating saline or synthetic contrast create microbubbles. These are very reflective,

Normal ranges for measures of systolic and diastolic function	
Echocardiography	
Fractional shortening (%)	28–44
Doppler	
Systolic velocity integral (cm)	15–35
Mitral valve E (cm/s)	44–100
Mitral valve A (cm/s)	20–60
E:A ratio	0.7–3.1
Tricuspid valve E (cm/s)	20–50
Tricuspid valve A (cm/s)	12–36
E:A ratio	0.8–2.9
Time intervals	
Mitral E deceleration time (ms)	139–219
Mitral A deceleration time (ms)	>70
Isovolumic relaxation time (ms)	54–98

Normal intracardiac dimensions (cm)		
	Men	Women
Left atrium	3.0–4.5	2.7–4.0
LV diastolic diameter	4.3–5.9	4.0–5.2
LV systolic diameter	2.6–4.0	2.3–3.5
IV septum (diastole)	0.6–1.3	0.5–1.2
Posterior wall (diastole)	0.6–1.2	0.5–1.1

Table 1. The approximate normal values for various cardiac structures. IV: interventricular; LV: left ventricular.

and when injected intravenously can be seen as opacification in the echo window. They are normally seen on the right side of the heart before being trapped and absorbed by the pulmonary capillaries, so have no route to the left side of the heart. The contrast created by the bubbles allows a left-to-right shunt to be seen as a jet "interrupting" the opacification of the right atrium. However, there is a theoretical risk of systemic air embolism with a right-to-left shunt.

Applications

Echo is the cheapest and least invasive method available for screening cardiac anatomy. Generalists most commonly request an echo to assess left ventricular (LV) dysfunction, to rule out the heart as a thromboembolic source, and to characterize murmurs. The approximate normal values for various cardiac structures are described in **Table 1**.

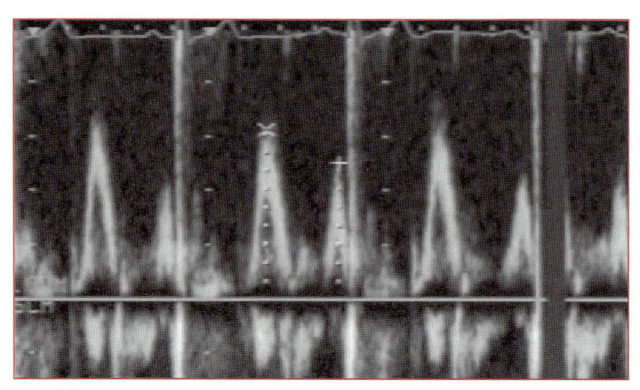

Figures 5. E and A waves representing mitral flow in a healthy heart (E>A).

Systolic dysfunction
LV systolic dysfunction is assessed using the ejection fraction (the percentage of the end diastolic volume ejected during systole). In most cases, this is estimated by eye from all the available echo views. A normal ejection fraction is 50%–80%, but values as low as 5% are compatible with life (end-stage heart failure).

The E/A ratio
When flow across the MV is assessed with PW Doppler, two waves are characteristically seen. These represent passive filling of the ventricle (early [E] wave) and active filling with atrial systole (atrial [A] wave). Classically, the E-wave velocity is slightly greater than that of the A wave (see **Figure 5**). However, in conditions that limit the compliance of the LV, two abnormalities are possible:

- reversal – in which the A wave is greater than the E wave. This indicates slow filling caused by older age, hypertension, left ventricular hypertrophy (LVH), or diastolic dysfunction
- exaggeration of normal – a tall, thin E wave with a small or absent A wave. This indicates restrictive cardiomyopathy, constrictive pericarditis, or infiltrative cardiac disease (eg, amyloidosis)

Diastolic dysfunction
A normal LV ejection fraction in the presence of the heart failure syndrome leads to a search for diastolic dysfunction. Typical echo findings in diastolic dysfunction are normal LV cavity size, thickened ventricle, and reversed E/A ratio.

Wall-motion abnormality
When ischemia occurs, contractile abnormalities of segments of the myocardium can be detected by echo prior to the appearance of electrocardiogram (ECG) changes or symptoms. Therefore, echo can be a valuable tool in the diagnosis of

Understanding the echocardiogram

	Mild or no aortic stenosis	Severe aortic stenosis
Area of effective orifice (cm^2)	>1	<0.6
Velocity across valve (m/s)	<3	>4
Gradient of pressure drop (mm Hg)	0–60	>60

Table 2. Echo characteristics of aortic stenosis.

both stable coronary artery disease (via stress echo) and acute myocardial infarction. In the former situation, it offers localization of the ischemic region where the ECG cannot; in the latter, it offers some measure of the extent of the infarct and a screen for complications, such as ventricular septal defect (VSD).

Valve assessment
Echo is the tool of choice for the assessment of valvular abnormalities.

Aortic stenosis
The etiology of aortic stenosis (AS) can be confirmed by the visualization of either a bicuspid valve or calcification. The severity of the stenosis can be estimated by measuring high-velocity flow across the valve by Doppler. This can be converted to an estimation of the pressure drop. In addition, the effective orifice area can be measured (see **Table 2**).

Aortic regurgitation
CFM is the most useful technique for detecting and quantifying the degree of regurgitation. The width of the regurgitant jet and of the slope of the decline in pressure gradient between the left ventricle and the aorta (which is reduced already compared with normal) are measured.

Mitral stenosis
With mitral stenosis (MS), as with AS, calcified, immobile MV leaflets can be demonstrated with 2D and M-mode echo. Anterior motion of the posterior MV leaflet in diastole (caused by commissural fusion) is characteristic in MS. Doppler demonstrates increased flow velocity and can be used to estimate the effective orifice area (see **Table 3**).

Mitral regurgitation
As with aortic regurgitation, mitral regurgitation is assessed using CFM. The severity of mitral regurgitation is commonly reported as the area of the regurgitant jet expressed as a percentage of the area of the left atrium.

	Mild mitral stenosis	Severe mitral stenosis
Area of effective orifice (cm^2)	>1.5	<1
Velocity across valve (m/s)	<2.5	>3

Table 3. Echo characteristics of mitral stenosis.

Mitral valve prolapse
The criteria for the diagnosis of MV prolapse (MVP) from an echo have changed over the years. Initial reports using the 4-chamber view suggested a population prevalence of almost 20%. However, a more accurate figure of approximately 5% results from stricter criteria. Most diagnose only on the basis of the parasternal long axis view. Some go so far as to suggest it is invalid to diagnose MVP on the 4-chamber view at all.

Paraprosthetic regurgitation
Although metal valves stop ultrasound completely, echo is a useful tool for studying prosthetic valve function. The TEE approach is often used.

Infective endocarditis
Echo is the key investigation in infective endocarditis and, although a low threshold for TEE is warranted by its higher detection rate, transthoracic echo can demonstrate vegetations in approximately 70% of cases (see Chapter 10, Infective endocarditis).

Embolic sources
The primary cardiac sources for embolism are:

- an akinetic ventricular segment
- an LV aneurysm
- the atrial appendage

These are best visualized with TEE.

Hypertrophic cardiomyopathy
Although hypertrophy is variable, echo remains the screening tool of choice in suspected cases. The classic features are asymmetrical hypertrophy of the interventricular septum and anterior movement of the MV in systole. LV function is normal, and there may be dynamic LV outflow tract obstruction.

Further reading

Chambers JB. *Clinical Echocardiography.* London: BMJ Books, 1995.

Feigenbaum HMD. *Echocardiography,* 5th edn. Philadelphia: Lea & Febiger, 1994.

Chapter 5

Coronary artery disease

Background

Coronary artery disease (CAD) is the most common cause of mortality in the developed world. It results from the collision of ancient genes with modern lifestyles: a hunter–gatherer lifestyle – with high daily energy expenditure and rare kills – favors a tendency to eat large quantities of high-calorie food when it is available. Such predispositions sit uneasily in a modern world with motorized transport and fatty snacks on every corner. Despite this, so-called "hardening of the arteries" was first described only in the 1700s, and it was not until the 1900s that a good description of myocardial infarction (MI) was forthcoming.

The term "coronary artery disease" encompasses a range of diseases that result from atheromatous change in coronary vessels. In the past, CAD was thought to be a simple, inexorable process of artery narrowing, eventually resulting in complete vessel blockage (and MI). However, in recent years the explanatory paradigm has changed because it was realized that a whole spectrum of coronary plaques exists – from stable (lipid-poor, thick fibrous cap) to unstable (lipid-rich, thin fibrous cap) (see **Figure 1**). When an unstable plaque ruptures – and the more unstable it is, the more likely it is to rupture – the subsequent release of prothrombotic and vasoconstrictive factors increases the likelihood of complete occlusion of the artery. It is the balance between the body's prothrombotic and thrombolytic pathways at the rupture site that determines the clinical outcome. Transient occlusion leads to ischemia and pain; permanent occlusion leads to transmural MI (see **Table 1**).

> **THROMBOSIS IN MYOCARDIAL INFARCTION**
> *The hypothesis that thrombosis plays a central role in myocardial infarction was first proposed by James Herrick in JAMA in 1912. This paper was the first to suggest that clots, rather than a slow accretion of plaque, are responsible for the complete occlusion that would often result in death. Importantly, he was the first to link symptoms in living patients with coronary artery disease, and to suggest that patients can survive complete blockage. These ideas were radical and new and (not surprisingly) no one believed him.*

Chapter 5

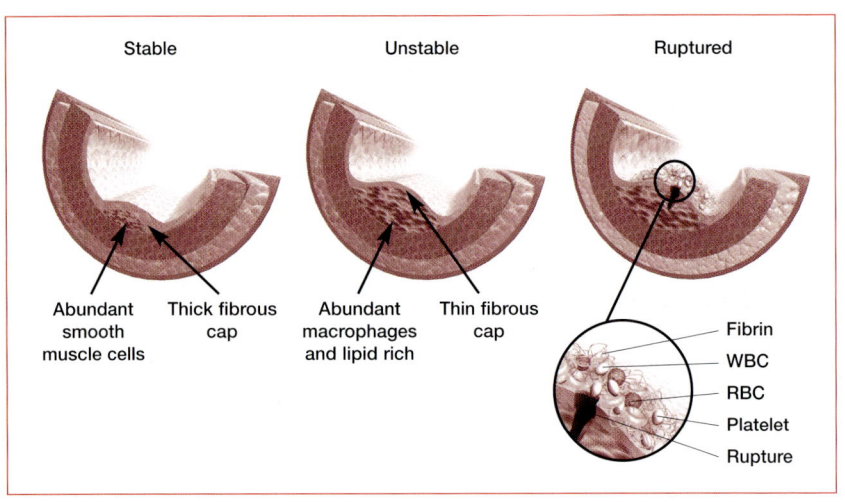

Figure 1. An atherosclerotic plaque consists of a core of dead foam cells (lipid-engorged macrophages and smooth muscle cells) covered by a fibrous cap (a region of the intimal layer that has become thickened as a result of medial smooth muscle cells depositing collagen and elastin fibers). The thickening artery wall of an atherosclerotic plaque gradually encroaches upon the luminal space and can eventually result in a restriction to blood flow. Unstable plaques, which are susceptible to rupture, are softer with a thinner fibrous cap. Plaque rupture triggers the formation of a blood clot, which can block the flow of blood through the artery. RBC: red blood cell; WBC: white blood cell.

Presentation	Vascular event
Stable angina	No plaque rupture, but symptomatic or limiting stable occlusion
Acute coronary syndromes (unstable angina/non-Q wave MI)	Plaque rupture with transient or incomplete occlusion
MI	Plaque rupture with complete occlusion and tissue necrosis

Table 1. Subgroups of coronary artery disease presentations. MI: myocardial infarction.

The establishment of these pathophysiological origins of CAD, together with the identification of improved clinical markers for ischemia and necrosis, has led to the proposal of a new (somewhat controversial) definition for acute MI: a rise and fall in troponin or the creatine kinase myocardial band fraction (CK-MB) (see "Markers of myocardial damage" section), plus at least one of the following:

- ischemic symptoms
- development of pathological Q waves on the electrocardiogram (ECG)
- ST-segment elevation or depression on the ECG
- coronary artery intervention (eg, angioplasty)

> **ANGINA PECTORIS**
> William Heberden defined angina pectoris in 1768 and provided a clear description of the familiar pain. However, it was Edward Jenner and Caleb Parry who linked this "disorder of the breast" with the "hardening" of the arteries that had been described by Giovanni Morgagni 7 years earlier.

Assessment

History and examination

History-taking is the most valuable technique for differentiating between the many causes of chest discomfort. The classic symptoms of angina are well known: a sensation of a constriction of the chest with variable levels of radiation to the neck, jaw, both arms, and occasionally to the epigastrium or through to the back. The pain is worse with exertion, especially in cold air; improved by rest and nitrates; and often follows a meal. Retrosternal pain in particular (often described by patients as "pressure") suggests that angina is the cause. Pains that are localized elsewhere, described as sharp or stabbing, or reproduced by palpation are much less likely to be cardiac in origin.

The term "unstable angina" encompasses a number of presentations, including pain that:

- occurs at rest
- lasts longer than 30 minutes
- is not relieved by several doses of sublingual nitrate
- is elicited over days or weeks by gradually smaller amounts of exertion (crescendo angina)

Examination of the cardiovascular system is mandatory in any patient reporting chest pain. Sweating, nausea, and vomiting are suggestive of MI, while complications of MI – such as heart failure (third heart sound and basal crackles) ventricular septal defect (VSD), harsh systolic murmur, or papillary muscle rupture – should be excluded.

Atypical chest pain

A common presentation in general practice is chest pain accompanied by an atypical history. In such cases, it is essential that the history is accurately established and documented. The most common noncardiac cause is dyspepsia. Although chest pain following a big meal could have a cardiac, gastroesophageal, or biliary origin, pain resulting from exercise is rarely biliary. It may be difficult to differentiate esophageal spasm from cardiac pain as they are both improved by nitrate. Other noncardiac causes to consider are musculoskeletal, pericardial, and pleural.

Chapter 5

Major independent risk factors	Predisposing risk factors	Possible risk factors
Cigarette smoking	Physical inactivity[a]	Fibrinogen
Hypertension	Obesity[a]	C-reactive protein
Elevated total and LDL cholesterol	Family history of premature coronary disease	Homocysteine
Low HDL cholesterol	Ethnicity	Elevated Lp(a)
Diabetes mellitus	Psychosocial factors	
Older age		

Table 2. American Heart Association guide to risk factors for coronary artery disease. HDL: high-density lipoprotein; LDL: low-density lipoprotein; Lp(a): lipoprotein little a. [a]These are classified as major by some bodies.

Other forms of angina include:

- variant angina (also known as Prinzmetal's angina), which causes an unpredictable pain – typically coming on at rest – and is associated with transient ST elevation on an ECG. It is thought to be due to coronary spasm and seems to be independent of atherosclerosis
- syndrome X – a condition in which the history is typical of coronary disease and there is ST depression on exercise, yet the coronary arteries are angiographically normal. It is thought to reflect small vessel disease and/or abnormal ventricular function
- dyspnea – angina can present as exertional dyspnea. Pay close attention to the pattern of onset and relief
- silent ischemia – diabetics, an important subgroup, can suffer from silent ischemia and even silent MI. Thus, even if there are no apparent symptoms of cardiac disease, a diabetic with an ECG abnormality should undergo stress testing and echocardiography to determine whether there is any indication for catheterization. One view is that all diabetics of greater than 5 years standing should be screened for cardiovascular disease

The key message is that a patient with an atypical history should always be referred for exercise electrocardiography (see "Investigations" section). In more than 90% of cases, the existence of coronary disease can be predicted accurately from the combined results of exercise ECG and their history.

Generalist management

Risk factors

Risk factor assessment and management are central to the care of cardiac patients. The major independent and predisposing risk factors (see **Tables 2** and **3**) should be documented for every patient, and it is useful to include them in every referral.

Lifestyle	Biochemical or physiological characteristics (modifiable)	Personal characteristics (nonmodifiable)
Diet high in saturated fat, cholesterol, and calories Tobacco smoking Excess alcohol consumption Physical inactivity	Elevated blood pressure Elevated plasma total cholesterol (LDL cholesterol) Low plasma HDL cholesterol Elevated plasma triglycerides Hyperglycemia/diabetes Obesity Thrombogenic factors	Older age Male gender Family history of CHD or other atherosclerotic vascular disease at early age (men <55 years, women <65 years) Personal history of CHD or other atherosclerotic vascular disease

Table 3. European Society of Cardiology table of lifestyles and characteristics associated with an increased risk of a future coronary heart disease (CHD) event. HDL: high-density lipoprotein; LDL: low-density lipoprotein.

Smoking
There are a wealth of products aimed at smoking cessation. Older products such as nicotine chewing gum have been replaced by nicotine patches and nicotine inhalers, and many products have been shown to have clear benefits in helping people to stop smoking. However, if someone is to succeed at giving up smoking, it is important that certain vital support mechanisms are in place before they attempt it:

- it is essential that the patients' families and partners are supportive
- patients should allocate a particular date and time to stop smoking. This should be a few weeks subsequent to the decision to stop, to allow time for planning and reflection
- patients should identify (and write down) the "at-risk" times when they envisage that temptation and craving will be greatest, for example with coffee or in a bar. They can then focus, in advance, on these situations and devise a way to avoid giving in
- on the allotted date, patients should remove all cigarettes and smoking materials from the house
- patients should keep diaries of their progress and report regularly to their doctor

Most people can stop smoking using these techniques. In cases where it is not successful, pharmacological help in the form of bupropion (Zyban) may be indicated. Helping patients to stop smoking is an extremely worthwhile endeavor. The risk tables (see **Figures 2** and **3**) show just how much there is to be gained by changing smoking status.

Chapter 5

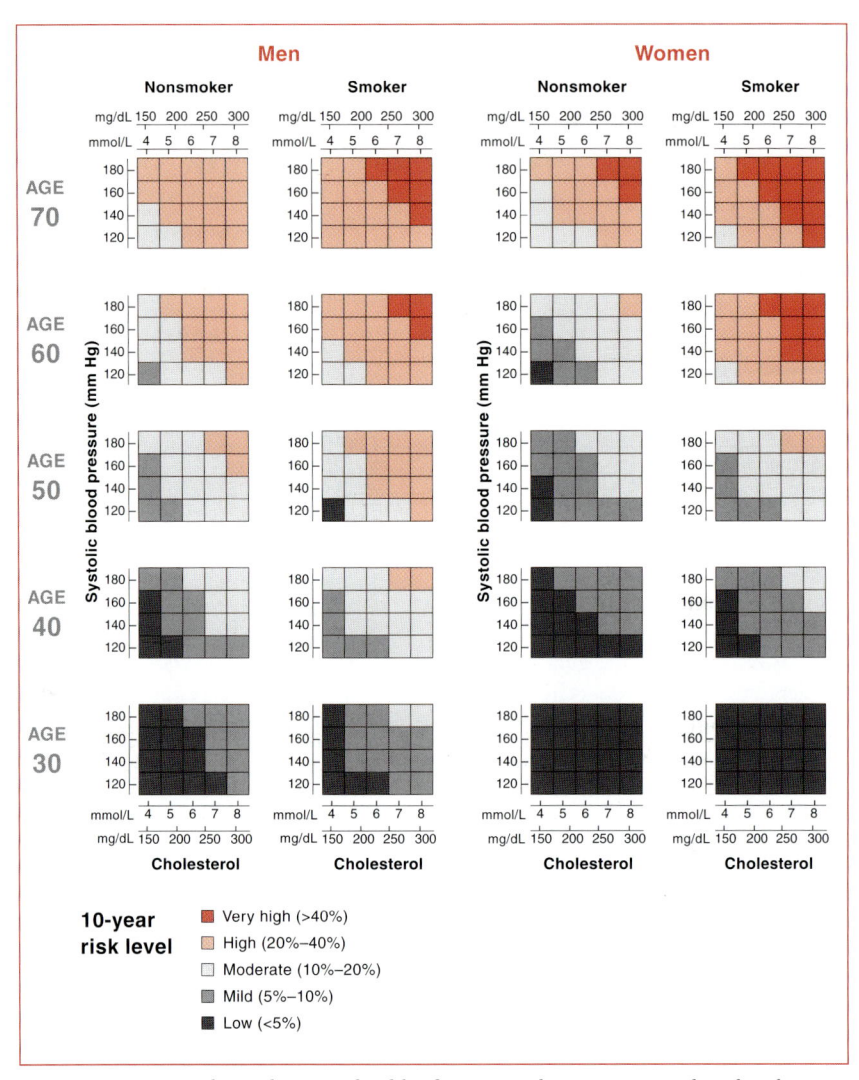

Figure 2. Coronary heart disease risk tables for men and women. Reproduced with permission from the European Society of Cardiology (Prevention of coronary heart disease in clinical practice. Recommendations of the Second Joint Task Force of European and other Societies on coronary prevention. *Eur Heart J* 1998;19:1434–503).

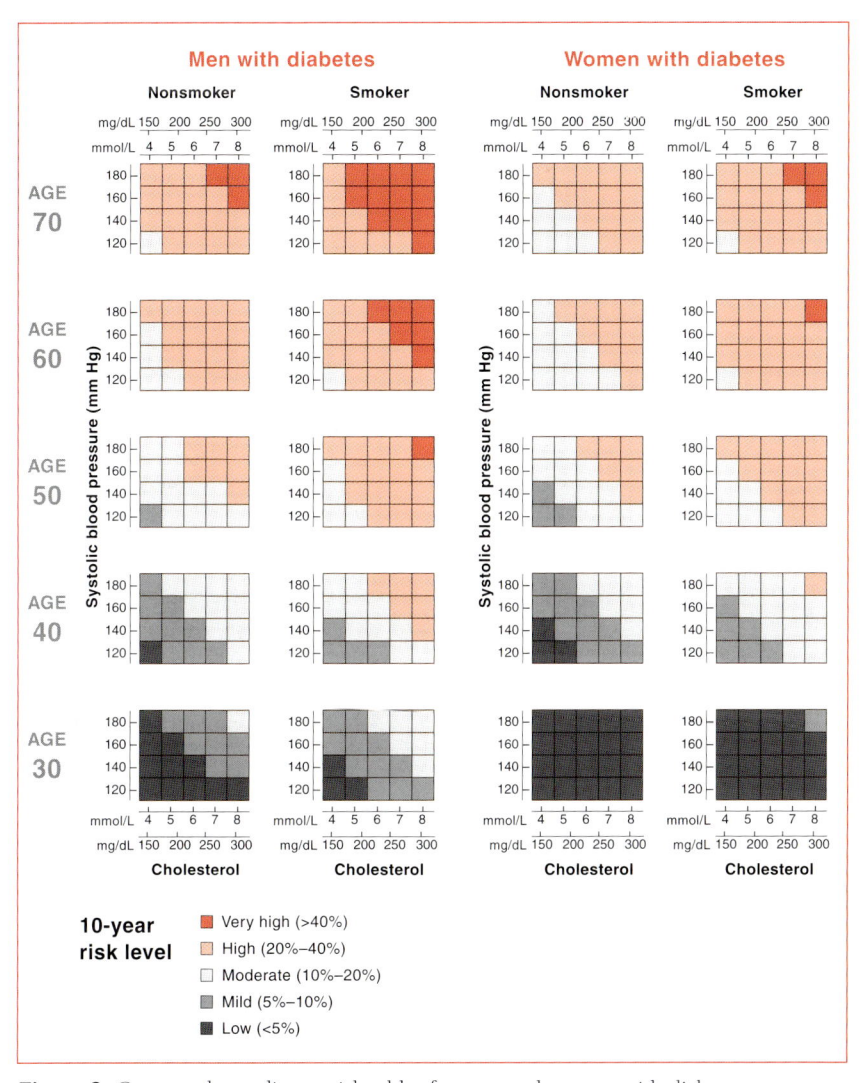

Figure 3. Coronary heart disease risk tables for men and women with diabetes. Reproduced with permission from the European Society of Cardiology (Prevention of coronary heart disease in clinical practice. Recommendations of the Second Joint Task Force of European and other Societies on coronary prevention. *Eur Heart J* 1998; 19:1434–503).

Chapter 5

Basic science

Exercise training exerts many beneficial changes at the cellular and molecular level. An exercise-induced increase in blood flow may exert its beneficial effects on vascular reactivity and structure through an increase in the elaboration of several endothelium-derived substances, such as nitric oxide, prostacyclin, and superoxide dismutase. Although prostacyclin may exert its antiatherogenic effects by inhibiting the uptake of cholesterol esters into macrophages or into smooth muscle cells, nitric oxide contributes strongly to the inhibition of monocyte adhesion, and inhibits platelet aggregation at much lower concentrations than those needed to inhibit adhesion, thereby allowing platelets to participate in the repair of the vessel wall, while at the same time preventing or limiting thrombus formation.

Flow also modulates the expression of numerous paracrine substances, including endothelial growth factors, matrix modulators, chemokines, and regulators of blood fluidity, all of which may participate in the beneficial effects of exercise-induced vascular remodeling and reactivity.

Finally, exercise-induced changes in flow also have other antiatherogenic effects. Endothelial cells exposed to shear stress elaborate less superoxide anion; this may in part be due to increased transcription of superoxide dismutase. There are also shear stress responsive elements in the promoter region of several adhesion molecules (eg, intercellular adhesion molecule) that may reduce their gene expression.

Diet
The central components of a healthy diet are well known: low in fat; low in salt; low in cholesterol; low in calories. In detail, patients should consume a diet high in fiber (>20 g/day), and low in fat (<10% of total amount of calories) and cholesterol (<300 mg/day). However, helping patients to achieve this is another matter. Dieticians and specialist nurses can give patients the advice and support they need to improve their diet.

Physical activity
It is very important that an increase in physical activity accompanies an improved diet and giving up smoking. Exercise can be an enjoyable undertaking for patients. It can help them to:

- improve their mood
- feel more energetic
- be less restricted in what they eat
- relax more
- sleep better
- take a break from their normal routine

With these benefits, it is surprising that anyone needs to be persuaded to exercise. Major bodies, led by the American College of Sports Medicine, recommend that patients exercise for 30 minutes on at least 3 days per week at a submaximal exercise intensity. However, exercise does not have to comprise formal exercise; it can include informal exercise, provided it is of adequate intensity. In this way, increases in physical activity can be absorbed into everyday life: for example, climbing the stairs instead of taking the elevator and walking to work instead of driving. In fact, walking, partly because it is so inefficient, is excellent exercise. Few people realize that walking a mile and running a mile use similar amounts of energy. Thus, there is no need for patients to join a gym (with all the expense that may be incurred) when daily brisk walking is ample exercise. Keeping a diary of their physical activity may help patients to sustain adequate amounts of daily exercise.

Submaximal aerobic exercise in angina
Many angina patients refrain from physical activity because they believe that the resulting pain is "dangerous". However, aside from its well-known benefits in risk reduction, exercise can be as effective as β-blockade in the management of stable angina. It has been associated with increased plaque stability and even slight plaque shrinkage. It is recommended that patients exercise for 30–45 minutes per day, 4–5 times a week.

Estimating risk
Formal risk estimation is aided by a standard set of tables that were developed using epidemiological data gathered over many years (see **Figures 2** and **3**). These tables are based on:

- gender
- age
- presence of diabetes
- smoking
- systolic blood pressure
- total cholesterol to high-density lipoprotein (HDL) ratio

Investigations
Electrocardiogram
The ECG is a vital tool for assessing patients in both stable and emergency situations. Nevertheless, generalists in primary care do not always have ready access to it. Any patient presenting with clear cardiac chest pain should undergo an ECG immediately or as soon as possible (preferably even before a history is taken) to identify whether they are at high risk, ie, ST segment change or new left bundle branch block (LBBB). This facilitates prompt referral when necessary and, for thrombolysis, a door-to-needle time of less than 30 minutes. However, the ECG

is not absolute – ST-segment elevation is present in only 50% of enzyme-confirmed MIs (see "Markers of myocardial damage" section).

Chest radiograph
A chest x-ray (CXR) may be used to help rule out aortic dissection in an acute presentation, although the gold standard is computed tomography (CT). Otherwise, it is rarely helpful. It should not be carried out on a routine basis.

Pharmacological management of angina
Stable disease is treated with aspirin and agents that offload or reduce the workload of the heart. Thus, standard medication for stable angina includes β-blockers, aspirin, and, if still symptomatic, long-acting nitrates.

Aspirin
The evidence for aspirin is so strong that it has to be part of the drug regimen of every patient with CAD. If aspirin is not tolerated, clopidogrel may be given instead. In cases in which warfarin (Coumadin) has to be administered (eg, coronary disease and atrial fibrillation), aspirin is usually omitted, since oral anticoagulation with an international normalized ratio (INR) of 3–4 has been shown to be safe and effective.

Oral long-acting nitrate
Nitrates are smooth muscle relaxants with the ability to vasodilate both the arteriolar and venous circulation. This leads to reductions in both preload (venous return) and afterload (blood pressure). However, nitrate-free periods are necessary to avoid tolerance.

Beta-blockers and calcium-channel blockers
Beta-blockers work by reducing the heart rate (lengthening diastole increases the time for coronary perfusion) and reducing the effects of catecholamine-mediated increases in cardiac workload. Calcium-channel blockers cause coronary artery dilation and subsequently decrease cardiac workload by reducing the contractility of myocardial smooth muscle cells. Calcium-channel blockers can be divided into rate-limiting (eg, verapamil, diltiazem) and nonrate-limiting (dihydropyridines, eg, amlodipine). Dihydropyridines are generally prescribed for hypertension, whereas the others tend to be used in cases of angina because of their ability to reduce the heart rate. However, verapamil should not be used with β-blockers, which block the action of sympathetic hormones (resulting in a lower heart rate and blood pressure) (see Chapter 6, Hypertension).

Potassium-channel openers

Potassium-channel openers, such as nicorandil, are a new class of agents for the treatment of angina. They exert both direct action on cardiac mitochondria and a nitrate-like effect. These are not yet available in the US.

Lipid-lowering agents

Lipids are insoluble in water. Hence, they are transported around the body as lipoproteins. Lipoproteins are made up of cholesterol, triglycerides, phospholipids, and protein. The major classes of lipoproteins (which vary in density, size, and triglyceride/cholesterol ratio) are:

- chylomicrons (the largest and least dense)
- very low-density lipoproteins (VLDLs)
- low-density lipoproteins (LDLs)
- HDLs

Lipids originate from two sources: endogenous lipids, synthesized in the liver, and exogenous lipids, ingested and processed in the intestine (see **Figure 4**).

Dietary cholesterol and triglycerides are packaged into chylomicrons in the intestine, before passing into the bloodstream via lymphatics. Chylomicrons are broken down by lipoprotein lipase (LPL) in the capillaries of muscle and adipose tissue to fatty acids, which then enter the cells. The chylomicron remnants, which have lost much of their triglyceride content, are taken up by the liver for disposal.

The liver synthesizes triglycerides and cholesterol, and packages them as VLDLs before releasing them into the blood. When VLDLs (which consist mainly of triglyceride) reach muscle and adipose blood vessels, their triglycerides are hydrolyzed by LPL to fatty acids. The fatty acids that are released are taken up by the surrounding muscle and adipose cells. During this process, the VLDLs become progressively more dense and turn into LDLs. While most of the resulting LDLs are taken up by the liver for disposal, some circulate and distribute cholesterol to the rest of the body tissues.

HDLs, which are also secreted from the liver and intestine, have the task of preventing lipid accumulation. They remove surplus cholesterol from tissues and transfer it to LDLs that return it to the liver.

To regulate cholesterol uptake, cells vary the expression of their LDL receptors. Elevated concentrations of lipid (hyperlipidemia) can lead to the development of atherosclerosis and CAD. VLDLs and LDLs are atherogenic lipoproteins, whereas HDL concentrations are inversely related to the incidence of CAD. Hence,

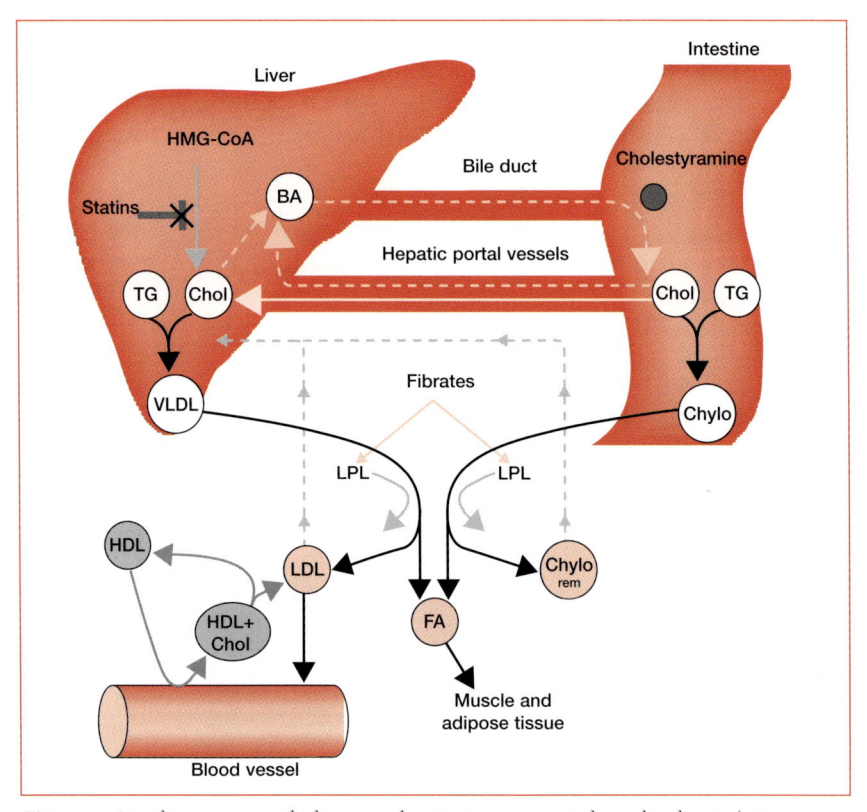

Figure 4. Lipid transport and pharmacotherapeutic agents in hyperlipidemia (see "Lipid-lowering agents" text). BA: bile acid; Chol: cholesterol; Chylo: chylomicron; Chylo rem: chylomicron remnant; FA: fatty acid; HDL: high-density lipoprotein; HMG-CoA: hydroxymethylglutaryl coenzyme A reductase; LDL: low-density lipoprotein; LPL: lipoprotein lipase; TG: triglyceride; VLDL: very low-density lipoprotein.

treatments for hyperlipidemia aim to reduce LDL levels and raise HDL levels. Pharmacotherapeutic options in hyperlipidemia include:

- statins, which inhibit hydroxymethylglutaryl coenzyme A reductase (HMG-CoA), the rate-limiting enzyme of cholesterol synthesis in the liver. A reduction in cholesterol synthesis causes the liver to increase the number of LDL receptors, reducing circulating concentrations of both cholesterol and triglyceride
- cholestyramine, which is a lipid-lowering drug that acts by sequestering bile acids in the gut, thus increasing the synthesis of bile acids from cholesterol
- fibrates, which reduce the level of VLDL by increasing the activity of the VLDL-hydrolyzing enzyme LPL

Guidelines for the use of lipid-lowering therapy have become more aggressive over the past few years following the results of major trials showing mortality benefit for the use of statins. Most guidelines recommend statin treatment for a patient with CAD with a 10-year risk that is greater than 20% (high risk) once a trial of dietary therapy has been unsuccessful. However, treatment can be cost effective with a 10-year risk of 10%. Recent trials have identified anti-inflammatory properties of statins and benefit even in patients with normal cholesterol levels. Dosage should be adjusted according to cholesterol levels. As part of secondary prevention, the following levels should be reached: total cholesterol, <200 mg/dL (5.2 mmol/L); HDL, >40 mg/dL (1 mmol/L); LDL, <100 mg/dL (2.6 mmol/L); triglyceride, <200 mg/dL (2.3 mmol/L).

Refer with confidence

Early management of stable coronary disease is mostly done in the community. Risk factor and stepwise pharmacological management of stable angina are appropriate. If there is any doubt about the diagnosis, a noninvasive test for coronary disease – such as an exercise ECG – should be carried out. Exercise ECG is increasingly carried out by generalists in primary care and hospitals. Pain that is resistant to medical therapy or crescendo symptoms warrants immediate presentation to an emergency room to rule out MI. The patient should then be referred to a cardiologist for further investigation, if needed. When referring patients who have had prior intervention, try to summarize the details of previous revascularization. For example:

- two-vessel disease (left anterior descending [LAD], circumflex artery)
- previous left internal mammary artery (LIMA) graft to LAD, percutaneous transluminal coronary angioplasty (PTCA) to right coronary artery (RCA)
- previous saphenous vein graft (SVG) to circumflex artery

Including this type of detail will greatly increase the usefulness of a referral letter.

Specialist management

Stable angina: assessment
Exercise electrocardiography
Exercise ECG is the mainstay test for the diagnosis of CAD. It is usually carried out on a treadmill, but bicycle exercise can also be used. The patient exercises according to a set protocol from rest to maximum exertion, which should be reached in 8–12 minutes. The protocol most commonly used was originally described by Robert Bruce and bears his name (see **Figure 5**). There are, however, good reasons to consider a protocol that is individualized for each patient. Diagnostic exercise

Chapter 5

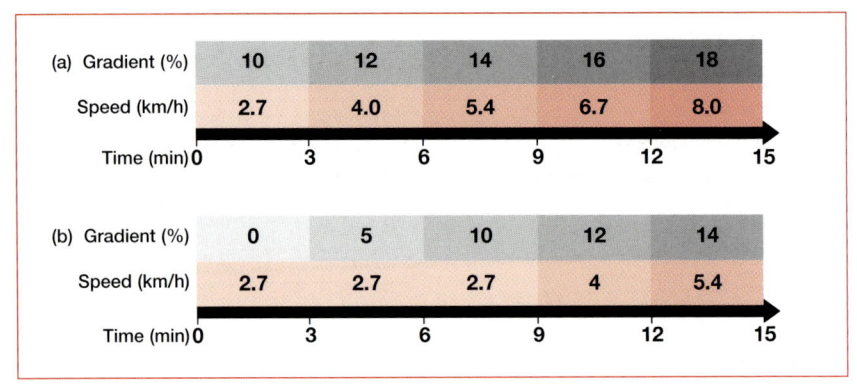

(a) Gradient (%)	10	12	14	16	18
Speed (km/h)	2.7	4.0	5.4	6.7	8.0
Time (min)	0	3	6	9	12	15

(b) Gradient (%)	0	5	10	12	14
Speed (km/h)	2.7	2.7	2.7	4	5.4
Time (min)	0	3	6	9	12	15

Figure 5. (a) The Bruce exercise protocol. The patient starts exercising at a speed of 2.7 km/h on a gradient of 10%. The workload is intensified every 3 minutes by increasing the speed and the incline of the treadmill, until the endpoint is achieved. (b) The modified Bruce exercise protocol is less intense to start with and is used to assess frailer patients, such as the elderly or those who have suffered a myocardial infarction.

tests focus predominantly on the ST segment, which must fall more than 1 mm from rest and be horizontal or downsloping to be significant. ST depression does not localize ischemia so it cannot reveal anything about a suspected coronary lesion, but it does enable a classification of mild, intermediate, or severe CAD to be made.

The exercise test is also useful for recording other variables, ie, work capacity; maximum heart rate and chronotropic incompetence; blood pressure rise and recovery; and heart rate recovery. Work capacity (presumably reflecting left ventricular [LV] function) and heart rate recovery are very strong prognostic indicators for CAD. Contraindications to exercise testing and reasons for stopping an exercise test are outlined in **Table 4**.

It is important to appreciate where the value of the exercise test lies:

- exercise ECG on its own has low sensitivity (<50%) but high specificity (>90%) – ie, it is very good at ruling disease in, but not good at ruling it out
- the meaning of the test results is significantly affected by the pretest probability of disease (see **Table 5**). For example, exercise-induced ST depression in a young woman with no risk factors is likely to be a false positive
- incorporating clinical and demographic information into the basic test result by calculating diagnostic "scores" can increase the sensitivity and specificity to >90% (see **Figure 6**)
- patients without a clear diagnosis from the exercise tolerance test should have another noninvasive test

Coronary artery disease

Contraindications to exercise testing	Reasons for stopping an exercise test
Unstable angina	Development of anginal symptoms
Left main stem disease	Fall >15 mm Hg or failure to increase systolic blood pressure
Acute myocarditis or pericarditis	
Untreated congestive cardiac failure	Arrhythmia development – ventricular in particular
Evidence of pyrexial or "flu"-like illnesses	An ST-segment depression of >2 mm in chest leads or >1 mm in limb leads
Severe aortic stenosis or HCM with marked outflow obstruction	
Dissecting aneurysm	
Adults with complete heart block	
Untreated severe hypertension	
LBBB (the test is nondiagnostic)	

Table 4. Contraindications to and reasons for stopping an exercise test. HCM: hypertrophic cardiomyopathy; LBBB: left bundle branch block.

Age (years)	Nonanginal chest pain		Atypical angina		Typical angina	
	Men	Women	Men	Women	Men	Women
30–39	4	2	34	12	76	26
40–49	13	3	51	22	87	55
50–59	20	7	65	31	93	73
60–69	27	14	72	51	94	86

Table 5. Pretest likelihood of coronary artery disease (CAD) in symptomatic patients according to age and sex – each value represents the percentage of patients found to have significant CAD on catheterization. Reproduced with permission from Lippincott Williams & Wilkins (Gibbons RJ, Chatterjee K, Daley J et al. ACC/AHA/ACP-ASIM Guidelines for the Management of Patients with Chronic Stable Angina: Executive Summary and Recommendations. *Circulation* 1999;99:2829–48).

A diagnostic algorithm for CAD is outlined in **Figure 7**. Most guidelines suggest the use of an alternative test if the preprobability is low. If the preprobability is high, exercise testing adds little in the way of diagnosis, but is useful for risk stratification. The primary role of exercise testing is where preprobability is intermediate.

Nuclear cardiology
Isotopes such as thallium-201 or technetium (Tc)-99m can be used to provide information on cardiac function.

Chapter 5

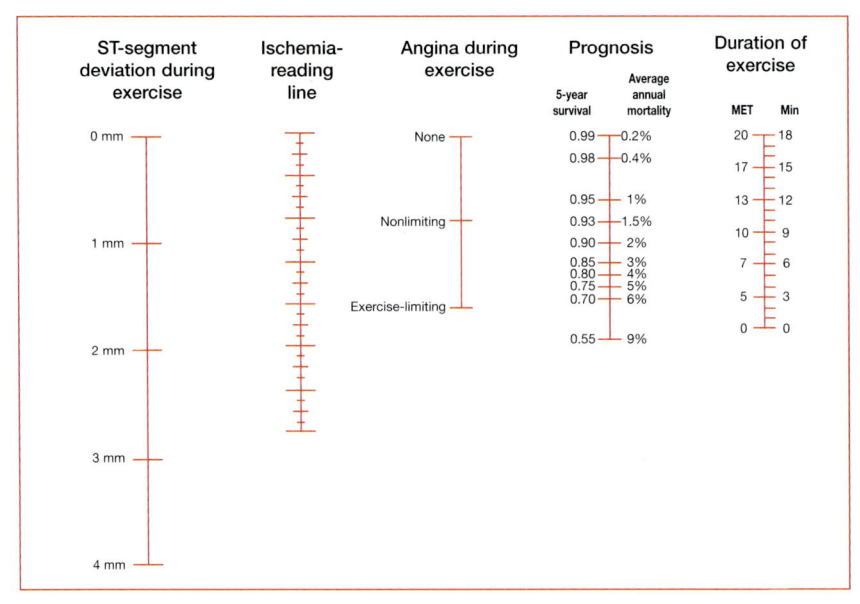

Figure 6. The Duke score, which is the most commonly used risk score, can be used for diagnosis as well as prognosis. To use this nomogram: determine (i) the maximum amount of downsloping or planar ST depression, and (ii) the type of angina during exercise. Connect these to give a point on the ischemia reading line. Then connect this point to the MET level (or duration of the Bruce protocol). Where this line dissects the prognosis line gives an estimate of risk. MET: metabolic unit – 1 MET equates to resting metabolic rate (typically 3.5 mL/kg/min).

Perfusion imaging is used to assess regional blood flow by comparing the relative distribution of isotope at rest and under conditions of stress. Stress is provided either by exercise or by pharmacological tools such as inotropes (eg, dobutamine) or vasodilators (eg, adenosine or dipyridamole). The isotope is injected at the peak of exercise and the image captured with a gamma camera. Rest images are usually achieved several hours later. The "exercise" and "rest" images are compared to identify perfusion defects that are either "fixed" (eg, the scar of an old MI) or "reversible" (ischemic disease). Thallium-201 has been the isotope of choice for many years, but more recently centers have been using Tc-99m-labeled compounds, such as sestamibi, which achieve a higher resolution from a lower dose of radiation. Single photon emission CT (SPECT) is a technique that employs a gamma camera head that rotates around the patient to provide three-dimensional images.

Isotopes are also used in ventriculography. Estimates of LV function arrived at using this imaging technique are more accurate and reproducible than those resulting from echo. Consequently, ventriculography is indicated in:

Coronary artery disease

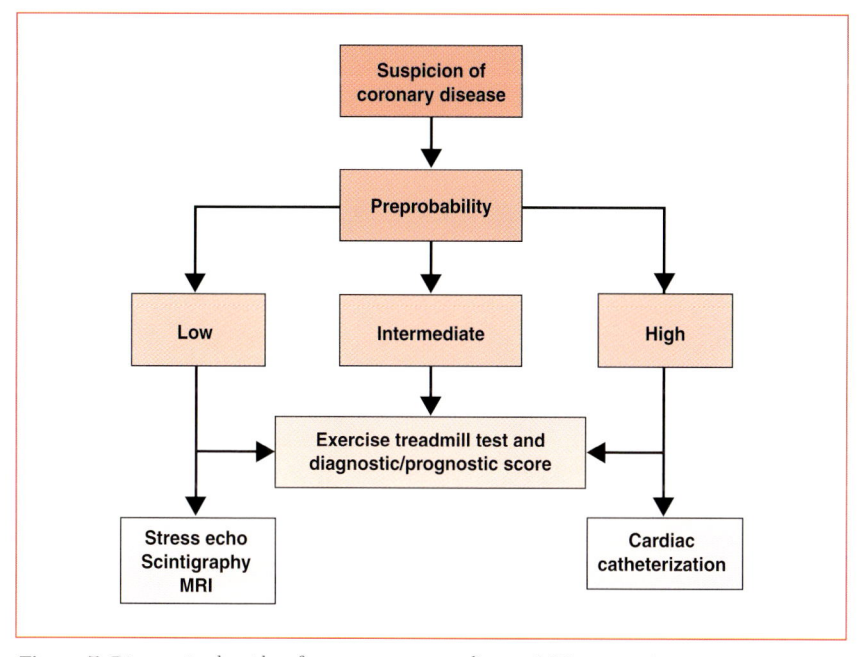

Figure 7. Diagnostic algorithm for coronary artery disease. MRI: magnetic resonance imaging.

- cardiomyopathy assessment
- pretransplant work-up
- any situation where accurate risk assessment is critical

Two types of protocol are used: equilibrium and first-pass. The former, which is more common, uses a sample of the patient's blood labeled with Tc-99m. Information is gathered from each heartbeat over the time of equilibration (a few minutes) then averaged to give the final reading. In the first-pass technique, a bolus of radionuclide is injected and information is gathered over a much shorter time with a fast gamma camera.

Stress echocardiography
Stress echo is gaining in popularity because it has:

- a higher predictive value than exercise ECG
- a lower cost and better safety profile than perfusion scintigraphy

Ultrasound is used to detect the difference in wall movement between ischemic and nonischemic myocardium (nonischemic myocardium moves less). Furthermore, the location of the wall-motion abnormalities enables the coronary disease pattern to be predicted – this is not possible from ST-segment depression on an exercise ECG. Stress echo is thus indicated when:

- LBBB is present on the resting ECG
- the exercise ECG is inconclusive for other reasons
- immobility or lung disease precludes the practical use of exercise as a cardiac stress (pharmacological stress echo only)

Stress echo can also provide information on stunned or hibernating myocardium. The former is myocardium that after a period of acute ischemia and reperfusion remains, for a time, hypokinetic at rest. Hibernating myocardium is a more chronic situation in which the blood flow of a segment is not adequate for function, yet is sufficient for it to remain viable. During periods of stress, these areas of myocardium "recover" and their viability can be detected as improvements (compared with at rest) in segmental contraction on exposure to low-dose pharmacological stress.

Stress echo is a useful technique in the hands of an experienced operator in a patient with a good echo window. Views can also be greatly improved by the use of a supine bicycle.

Electron beam computed tomography
This is a new technique that relies on imaging calcium in coronary lesions. It can quantify the "atherosclerotic burden" in the form of a calcium score to give an estimate of risk or to monitor the effect of, for example, lipid-lowering therapy. However, there is some doubt over how much information this measure adds to standard risk factors. Furthermore, vulnerable plaque often does not contain much calcium. The "holy grail" is a test that can locate and quantify "vulnerable" plaque, but this has not yet been found.

Magnetic resonance imaging
Most cardiologists agree that the future of noninvasive imaging of the heart lies with MRI. This technology can fulfill many of the functions of traditional tests and in most cases improve on them:

- cardiac anatomy and morphology can be assessed with a high degree of spatial resolution using "black-blood" imaging
- in cine mode (like two-dimensional echo), resolutions can be achieved that are significantly greater than those obtained with ultrasound and good views can be imaged and processed in under 30 seconds
- LV function – including under exercise/pharmacological stress – can be achieved with a single breath-hold and the circumferential shortening calculated

- wall-motion abnormalities can be assessed using tagging techniques
- perfusion imaging can be carried out with a single breath-hold and two R–R intervals

In fact, the only technique that is still some way from routine clinical application is magnetic resonance angiography (MRA) of the coronary vessels (larger vessel MRA has been possible for some time). However, as new technology moves the field forward, this is likely to become more attainable, and with it the tempting prospect of cross-sectional imaging and plaque characterization.

Stable angina: treatment
Cardiac catheterization
Since cardiac MRI is still only available in the bigger centers, coronary artery catheterization remains the diagnostic gold standard in CAD. As the conduit for coronary intervention, its position is also safe from advances in imaging technology. Catheterization can also be used in a variety of settings aside from CAD, such as ventricular dysfunction, valve disease, detection and quantification of shunts, and other congenital and acquired structural abnormalities.

The basic procedure of PTCA involves cannulation of the femoral artery, with manipulation of a catheter over a guide wire to the site of stenosis. Dye is injected into each coronary artery in turn to assess flow. Flow is graded using a system first put forward by the TIMI (Thrombolysis in Myocardial Infarction) investigators (see **Table 6**). In balloon angioplasty a balloon is inflated (using the image-enhancing contrast dye) to compress the atheroma and dilate the artery (see **Figure 8**). Until recently, this was the intervention of choice. However, balloon angioplasty has a restenosis rate of 30% over 6 months and a high rate of coronary artery dissection. Consequently, the use of coronary artery stents (see **Figure 8**), which have lower rates of restenosis and artery dissection, has become common practice. These are deployed using a balloon. Most recent work has focussed on drug-eluting stents (which elute anti-inflammatory or anti-proliferative agents), which seem dramatically to reduce the incidence of restenosis.

PIONEERS
In 1929, Werner Forssmann – a German cardiologist – went against the express advice of his boss and, with the help of a nurse, inserted a catheter through an arm vein into his own heart. This was the first time a human heart had ever been catheterized. He saw the successful catheterization images on a fluoroscope screen – only by using a mirror. A pioneer of cardiology, he published his paper in Klinische Wochenschrift *in 1929 and, although he catheterized only one patient's heart, he went on to catheterize his own heart another eight times.*

Contrast flow	TIMI grade
Prompt anterograde flow and rapid clearing	3
Slowed distal filling but full opacification of distal vessel	2
Small amount of flow but incomplete opacification of distal vessel	1
No contrast flow	0

Table 6. System (devised by the TIMI [Thrombolysis in Myocardial Infarction] investigators) used to grade the flow of contrast dye that has been injected into coronary arteries during percutaneous transluminal coronary angioplasty.

Other, less common percutaneous techniques include radioactive stents and atherectomy (where the atheroma is physically removed from the artery).

Insertion of a metal object into an artery is a prothrombotic event. Hence, stenting is carried out in conjunction with antithrombotic therapy. Infusional antithrombotic agents (eg, abciximab – see below) are used as an adjunct during angioplasty while oral antiplatelet agents, such as ticlopidine and clopidogrel, are used for 1 month post stent. (However, ticlopidine has been plagued by problems of bone marrow suppression.)

Abciximab – a chimeric murine–human Fab[1] fragment monoclonal antibody – and the small molecule inhibitors tirofiban and eptifibatide are members of a new class of antithrombotics. These agents function by inhibiting glycoprotein (GP)IIb/IIIa, a receptor abundant on platelets. When platelets are activated, this receptor binds fibrinogen and von Willebrand factor, leading to platelet aggregation.

The benefit from these agents almost certainly relates to microembolization since:

- there is good evidence from autopsy studies that, following spontaneous or instrumented coronary plaque disruption, small aggregates of platelets, cholesterol, or other plaque material can be found in distal microvessels
- it has been demonstrated, using filter devices and contrast echo, that microembolization is common following percutaneous coronary intervention (PCI) and is almost certainly the basis of "no reflow" – when perfusion is limited following PCI despite adequate restoration of flow in the infarct-related artery
- troponin levels, which are thought to be a sensitive marker for this type of damage, are elevated following approximately 40% of procedures. (Note that, in unstable angina, the benefit of GPIIb/IIIa inhibitors is not limited to those with elevated troponin levels.)

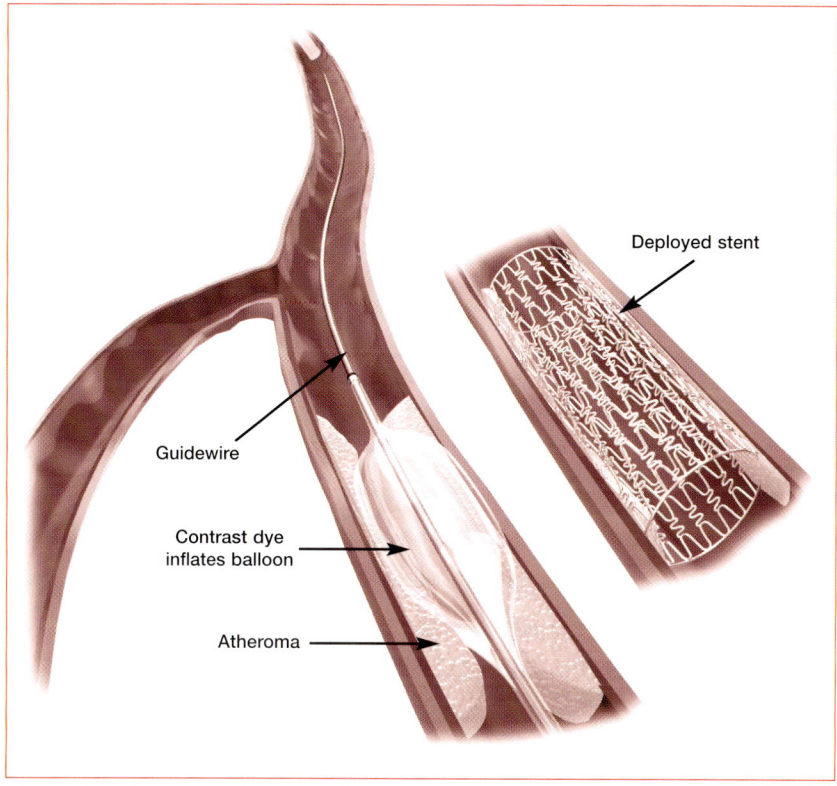

Figure 8. Balloon angioplasty is used to compress atherosclerotic narrowing and dilate the artery. A balloon is directed over a guidewire to the site of stenosis where it is inflated (by contrast medium) to push open the narrowing or deploy the stent.

Overall, complications from cardiac catheterization are relatively rare (totaling ~5%). They include:

- contrast allergy response (very rare due to modern dyes)
- local hemorrhage from puncture sites with subsequent thrombosis
- false aneurysm or arteriovenous (AV) malformation
- vasovagal reactions
- coronary dissection
- aortic dissection or ventricular perforation
- air or atheroma embolism, which can occur in either the coronary or other arterial circulations with consequent ischemia or stroke
- ventricular dysrhythmias, which are seen and may even cause death in the setting of left main stem disease

Chapter 5

> **THE FIRST HUMAN CORONARY ANGIOGRAM**
> *The first human coronary angiogram was, in fact, carried out by mistake by Mason Sones of the Cleveland Clinic in Ohio, USA, in 1958. Carrying out a standard LV angiogram, he paused – leaving the catheter in the aorta – to have a midprocedure smoke with his second operator. He returned, and relying on a pressure reading rather than direct visualization to determine the position of the catheter, he injected the RCA instead of the left ventricle. Realizing the mistake immediately from the outline of the RCA on the fluoroscope screen, he rapidly removed the catheter – just as his patient arrested. Hesitating, with scalpel in hand prepared for open chest defibrillation, he noticed the rhythm was asystole and not ventricular fibrillation. Thinking he might be able to help clear the dye without resorting to direct application of the paddles onto the myocardium, he pounded his patient's chest shouting "Cough! Cough!" Perhaps it was a cough, or maybe the precordial thump, or perhaps even its repeated application[a] that restarted the patient's heart, but certainly the fact that the patient recovered was the spark that ignited a revolution in diagnostic medicine.*
> ([a]Presaging CPR – a technique not practiced for several years subsequently.)

Overall mortality rates are quoted at less than one in 1,000 cases, but this increases to one in 100 for higher risk cases.

Coronary artery bypass grafting

Coronary artery bypass grafting (CABG) is the technique of choice for three-vessel disease with depressed LV function and left main stem coronary disease. However, since coronary interventions have become much more sophisticated some studies have shown equal benefit from percutaneous treatment as compared with surgical treatment in patients with three-vessel disease. During surgery, the patient undergoes sternotomy followed by heart–lung bypass and cardiac arrest. A portion of the saphenous vein is dissected from the leg, reversed (to orientate the venous valves in the appropriate direction), and attached proximally to the aortic root and distally to the coronary artery (see **Figure 9**). The LIMA, which originates from the left subclavian artery, can also be used as a conduit. It is disconnected at its distal end only and the cut end is connected to the LAD. In the same way, the right internal mammary artery (RIMA) can be connected to the RCA. A clear benefit of LIMA/RIMA CABG is improved graft patency, both perioperatively and in the long term (10 years). Other arteries that can be used include the radial and the gastroepiploic.

Due to the risks of heart–lung bypass – such as postbypass cognitive deficit – some centers now practice beating heart surgery. In this procedure the heart is not arrested: the section of the heart that is to be operated on is stabilized locally by the "suckers" (vacuum-operated suction clamps) of a device known as an octopus. Another technique is minimally invasive bypass, which uses small incisions and LIMA grafts.

Coronary artery disease

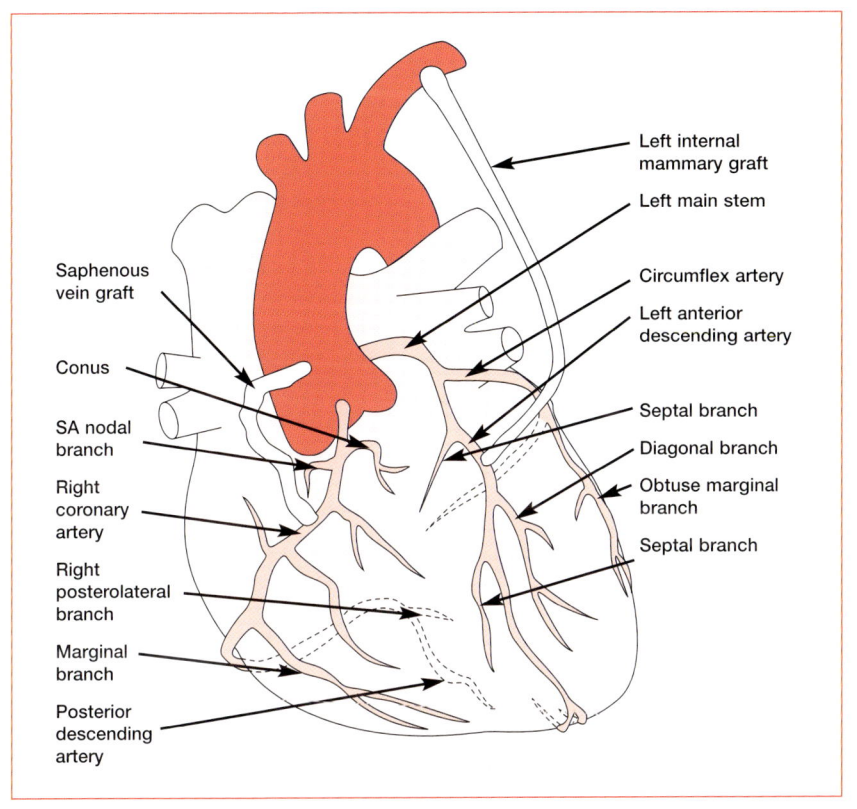

Figure 9. Sites of heart bypass grafting: a saphenous vein graft and a left internal mammary artery graft are shown.

Evidence base

With these rapid advances in both surgical and percutaneous techniques, much of the evidence base is out of date. For example, there are no definitive data indicating that angioplasty saves lives in stable CAD. Previous trials have shown that CABG can benefit outcome in: symptomatic, significant left main stem disease; symptomatic proximal three-vessel disease; and two-vessel disease including the proximal LAD. Patients with moderately impaired LV function benefit more from CABG than those with poor LV function, who have greater operative mortality (overall mortality is around 2.8%, but rises to 3.7%–12% for an emergency procedure).

Most cardiologists believe that new trials will demonstrate a mortality benefit for coronary stenting, possibly for three-vessel disease and perhaps even over and above that of bypass.

Marker	Initial rise	Peak	Return to normal	Notes
Troponin I/T	2–4 h	10–24 h	5–10 d	Troponin I and T are sensitive and specific markers (unlike troponin C). Their blood level clearly relates to risk and thus they represent a powerful tool for risk stratification
Creatine kinase[a]	3–4 h	10–24 h	2–4 d	CK-MB is the main cardiac isoenzyme
Lactate dehydrogenase	10 h	24–72 h	14 d	Myocardium mainly has LDH1
Myoglobin	1–2 h	4–8 h	24 h	Convenient early marker due to availability of assay, but not cardiac specific
Heart fatty-acid binding proteins	1.5 h	5–10 h	24 h	Undergoing evaluation

Table 7. Timescales for the variation in levels of markers for myocardial damage. CK-MB: creatine kinase myocardial band fraction; LDH1: lactate dehydrogenase 1.
[a]Creatine kinase has three isoenzymes, of which CK-MB is the most cardiac specific. However, other organs also possess this enzyme in small quantities. It has been suggested that a CK-MB/CK ratio of over 2.5 is very specific for myocardial infarction in the context of chest pain. However, even this is inaccurate in situations of significant acute or chronic skeletal injury, where CK levels are also high.

Acute coronary syndromes: assessment

Risk assessment is the key to in-hospital management of acute coronary syndromes (ACS). Patients with ST elevation need to be considered immediately for thrombolysis or acute intervention. Other patients should be closely monitored (preferably in a coronary care unit) if they have risk factors, previous infarction, poor ventricular function, and changing ST segments. In this situation, the key investigation is the measurement of cardiac enzymes.

Markers of myocardial damage

A number of markers for not only infarction, but also noninfarct ischemia, are now available. The transaminases aspartate aminotransferase (AST) and alanine aminotransferase (ALT) no longer offer any advantage over the other markers and in fact often cause false-positive results. Timescales of the variation in levels of the most commonly used markers for myocardial damage are outlined in **Table 7** and **Figure 10**. Of the markers in **Table 7**, troponin I or T are the most specific and sensitive markers to rule acute MI out or in.

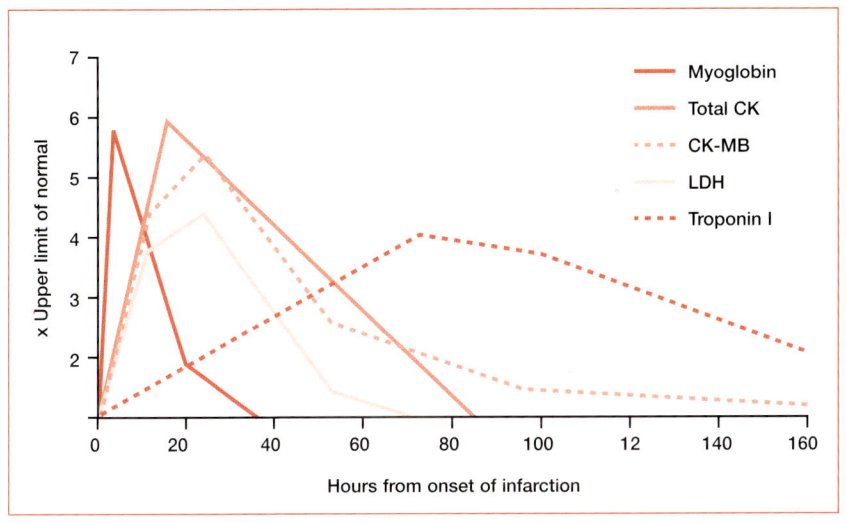

Figure 10. Appearance of cardiac markers in the blood after onset of symptoms. CK: creatine kinase; CK-MB: creatine kinase myocardial band fraction; LDH: lactate dehydrogenase.

Acute coronary syndromes: treatment
Pharmacological agents
The first-line treatment of any ACS is oxygen, aspirin, heparin, and β-blockade. Clopidogrel is an alternative to aspirin and diltiazem is an alternative to β-blockade. Low molecular-weight heparins have advantages over heparin, such as:

- simple administration
- better bioavailability
- no requirement for monitoring
- enhanced antifactor Xa activity
- lower rates of heparin-induced thrombocytopenia (HIT)

Nitrates can be given intravenously for closer control of pain, unless there is hypotension or suspicion of a posterior infarction that needs higher filling pressures. Tolerance to nitrates occurs very quickly (24–36 hours) so the quicker the infusion can be weaned, the better. Opiate analgesia is also used for pain. In both cases, there may be benefit from GPIIb/IIIa inhibitors (see above). Patients with positive troponin levels should undergo immediate catheterization. Otherwise, patients should rest until they are pain-free. After 48 hours without pain, patients should undergo cardiac catheterization.

Chapter 5

Myocardial infarction
If MI is confirmed by history and ST elevation (1 mm in limb leads, 2 mm in chest leads, or new LBBB) or elevated troponin plus either of these, the patient must quickly be taken to the catheterization laboratory. If this facility is not available, the doctor should immediately: (1) rule out contraindications to thrombolysis (see "Thrombolysis" section) and (2) arrange for analgesia and thrombolysis to be set up, before (3) completing the history and examination.

Primary PTCA
Recently – primarily due to improvements in devices, adjunctive therapy (GPIIb/IIIa inhibitors), and user experience – in cases of acute MI, the superiority of PTCA over thrombolysis alone has become clear. Most lesions (80%) are suitable for PTCA, particularly if they are discrete, proximal, uncalcified, subtotally occluded, without thrombus, and away from the side branches or divisions of a vessel. As such, primary PTCA is the procedure of choice for patients within 12 hours of the onset of MI symptoms. Current evidence suggests that patients of less than 75 years with cardiogenic shock (occurring within 36 hours of MI) benefit most from primary PTCA (within 18 hours of onset of shock) in an appropriate center with experienced personnel. In cases of poor LV function, intra-aortic balloon pumping (see Chapter 7, Heart failure) is useful in the setting of proximal LAD or mainstem stenting.

Thrombolysis
Thrombolysis is given as an infusion of (typically) streptokinase or tissue plasminogen activator (tPA) over 30 minutes to 1 hour, depending on the protocol. Aspirin and (intravenous) β-blocker should also be given acutely. Thrombolysis is beneficial up to 12 hours after the onset of pain, but may be given up to 24 hours afterwards in the context of continuing pain or a deteriorating condition.

The choice of thrombolytic agent is controversial. tPA and similar recombinant agents are still from 5- to 7-times more expensive than streptokinase and thus only tend to be used in the following situations:

- where streptokinase has been administered previously
- where recent proven streptococcal throat infections have occurred
- in cases of hypotension

However, even with large anterior MI in younger patients presenting within 4 hours (a situation where tPA is often recommended first-line), the absolute added mortality benefit is only 1% above streptokinase.

Intracranial hemorrhage (ICH) can be an important complication of thrombolysis. Since heparin is associated with an increased risk of ICH (streptokinase treatment has a lower rate of ICH when it is administered without heparin), there is particular concern with respect to the administration of tPA (as it is usually given with heparin) to hypertensive patients above 65 years of age who are less than 70 kg in weight. Partly as a result of these concerns, several centers have explored the use of low-dose thrombolytic treatment in combination with GPIIb/IIIa inhibition. The results of these trials have been encouraging.

Recanalization is achieved following thrombolysis in approximately 70% of cases (compared with 15% of cases without thrombolysis). As this leaves a significant minority needing further attention, all patients should be reviewed 2 hours following thrombolysis. Rethrombolysis or coronary intervention should be considered if there is no resolution in the ST segment.

There are few absolute contraindications to thrombolysis and risks must be weighed against benefits in each individual case, particularly in the face of a large anterior infarct in a patient where access to primary PTCA is unavailable. However, there are some absolute contraindications and some notable relative contraindications.

Absolute contraindications are:

- suspected aortic dissection (demands urgent CT, which is the gold standard, MRI, or transesophageal echo)
- active internal bleeding or uncontrollable external bleeding (excluding menses)
- recent head trauma (<2 weeks)
- intracranial neoplasms
- history of proven hemorrhagic stroke or cerebral infarction within 12 months
- untreated diabetic hemorrhagic/proliferative retinopathy
- BP >180/110 mm Hg uncontrolled (reduce with nitrates, β-blockade, angiotensin-converting enzyme inhibitors)

Relative contraindications are:

- pregnancy
- traumatic prolonged CPR
- anticoagulation or INR >1.8
- bleeding disorders
- recent surgery (within 3 weeks)
- probable intracardiac thrombus (eg, atrial fibrillation with mitral stenosis)
- active peptic ulcer

Chapter 5

> ## Basic science
>
> Atherosclerosis is initiated by a combination of circulating factors, such as cholesterol, and hemodynamic forces (common sites for atherosclerosis are areas where arteries branch). LDL and circulating leukocytes penetrate the arterial wall at regions of high shear stress (turbulent flow). In its atherogenic oxidized form, LDL enters macrophages, converting them to foam cells in the process. Oxidized LDL also enhances the growth factor-mediated migration of monocytes and smooth muscle cells to the intima, where the latter differentiate to form the fibrous cap of the mature atherosclerotic plaque. **Figure 11** shows the layers of a vessel wall.
>
> As a result of our understanding of these processes, there is much experimental interest in factors that contribute to the attraction and adhesion of leukocytes (chemokines and adhesion molecules), the receptors that modulate LDL uptake (scavenger receptors), enzymes that degrade the cap (matrix metalloproteinases), and protective species (such as nitric oxide). With inflammation a central component of our current appreciation of atherosclerosis, there is much interest in circulating markers (such as C-reactive protein) and pharmaceutical interventions that decrease inflammation (aspirin and statins).

Arrhythmia
Reperfusion arrhythmias are common in the first 2 hours following thrombolysis. In addition to ensuring that plasma potassium is above 4.5, intravenous amiodarone and therapeutic-dose magnesium are indicated for sustained ventricular tachycardia or in ventricular fibrillation as adjuncts to defibrillation. Amiodarone is usually given via a central line, but can also be administered via a large antecubital cannula, although the latter has a slightly higher risk of local necrosis. Arrhythmias occurring more than 48 hours after an acute MI are associated with a worse prognosis and should be investigated further by coronary angiography to rule out hemodynamically relevant coronary stenoses, and electrophysiological studies to rule out scar-tissue substrate.

Other therapy
Glycemic control should be optimized in all diabetic patients, preferably with the use of sliding-scale insulin.

Oral inotropes should be avoided since almost all randomized trials have shown an increased mortality over placebo.

Angiotensin-converting enzyme inhibitors and β-blockers are given within the first 24 hours post-MI (in the absence of hypotension or other specific contraindications). However, although there is clear evidence for the benefit of each

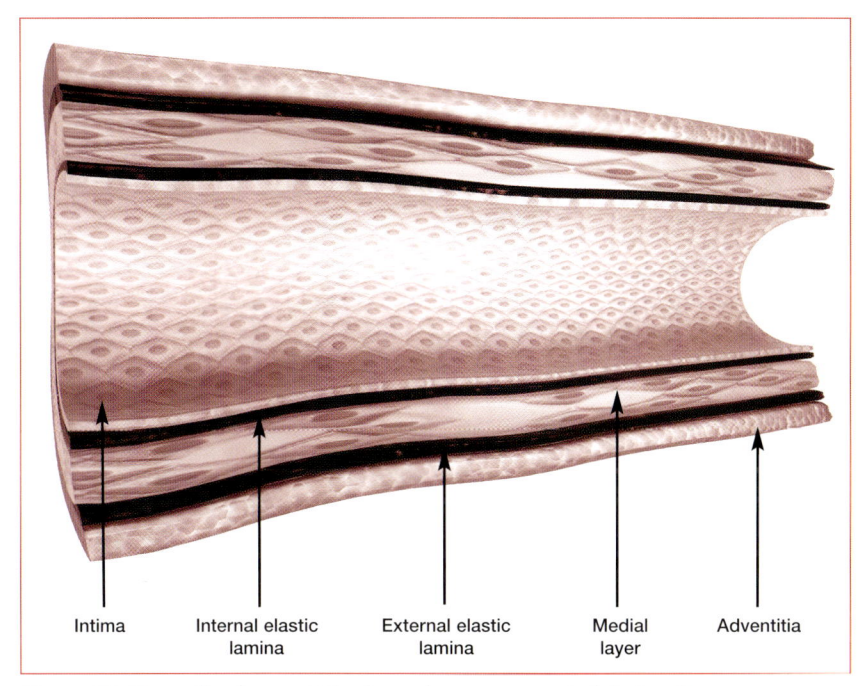

Figure 11. The walls of normal blood vessels are composed of distinct layers: the intima is the innermost layer. It consists of a single layer of endothelial cells lining the vessel, supported by a layer of connective tissue. The media is composed of smooth muscle cells and is sandwiched between the internal and external elastic laminae. The adventitia is the outermost layer and consists mostly of collagen fibers that protect the blood vessel.

agent individually, there are few data on their effect when used in combination. Until further data are available, both should be given together.

Short-acting calcium-channel blockers of the dihydropyridine type are contraindicated in acute MI. The longer-acting dihydropyridines may reduce reinfarction in patients with a first non-Q-wave infarction or inferior infarction in the absence of LV dysfunction and pulmonary edema. However, their benefit over aspirin and β-blockade in the context of MI is unclear.

Although warfarin provides no general benefit, in those patients with mural LV thrombus following a large acute anterior MI, it can reduce the overall rate of cerebrovascular complications (2%–3%) by more than half. Thus, it is recommended for up to 6 months following infarction, or longer if the thrombus is still nonlaminar on echo.

Chapter 5

Refer with confidence

Practices vary enormously from center to center, but it is still common for hospital generalists to manage non-ST elevation, low-risk ACS, and even MI where no facilities for intervention are available. In these situations, the most common scenarios for referral to cardiology would be:

- recurrent pain following proven MI
- unstable pain that refuses to settle
- recurrent episodes of atypical pain with no ECG change or enzyme rise

Cardiac rehabilitation

Although the general phenomenon of MI has been recognized for about 100 years, for the first 70 years our approach to its treatment was diametrically opposite to that which we now propose. Complete immobilization for anything from 4 to 8 weeks – even to the point where patients were fed, washed, and shaved – was thought to help the heart to form a firm scar. Exercise was thought to increase the risk of ventricular aneurysm, cardiac rupture, congestive heart failure, and sudden death.

How bold then were the early pioneers, such as Terry Kavanagh at the Toronto Rehab center, who in 1973 entered seven post-MI patients for the Boston Marathon (all seven finished). Not long after that, as the medical profession gained confidence in this new-found approach, the *Journal of Cardiac Rehabilitation* was founded by Mike Pollock and Victor Froelicher, and other pioneers were soon taking the field forward. Today, controlled trials have demonstrated that cardiac rehabilitation is not only safe and saves lives (25% reduction in mortality at 3 years), but is more cost-effective than other post-MI treatment interventions, such as thrombolytic therapy, coronary bypass surgery, and cholesterol-lowering drugs (though less cost-effective than smoking cessation programs).

Effective cardiac rehabilitation is multilayered and involves permanent lifestyle changes – such as the incorporation of regular physical activity into everyday life – to improve the risk profile. The many components of rehabilitation are outlined in **Table 8**. Programs are usually run by specialist nurses and physiologists, together with a cardiologist. However, in the absence of a local formal program, most of the components can be managed in the community. The potential benefits are enormous. The dramatic effect of cardiac rehabilitation is thought to be due to improvements in lipid profile, endothelial function, body composition, autonomic tone, fibrinolysis, and psychological well-being.

Elements of a cardiac rehabilitation program
Initial evaluation • medical history and examination • ECG • risk assessment • goal setting
Low-fat diet: a diet high in fiber (>20 g/day), and low in fat (<10% of total amount of calories) and cholesterol (<300 mg/day)
Management of lipid levels
Management of hypertension
Cessation of smoking
Weight reduction: body mass index <25 kg/m^2
Management of diabetes
Psychosocial management • identify depression, anxiety, social isolation, anger, and hostility • stress reduction
Activity counseling and exercise training • specific individualized aerobic and resistance training schedule, ie, 30 min/day on at least 3 days a week

Table 8. Elements of a cardiac rehabilitation program.

Further reading

Ashley EA, Myers J, Froelicher V. Exercise testing in clinical medicine. *Lancet* 2000;356:1592–7.

Balady GJ, Ades PA, Comoss P et al. Core components of cardiac rehabilitation/secondary prevention programs: A statement for healthcare professionals from the American Heart Association and the American Association of Cardiovascular and Pulmonary Rehabilitation Writing Group. *Circulation* 2000;102:1069–73.

Braunwald E, Antman E, Beasley J et al. ACC/AHA Guidelines for the management of patients with unstable angina and non-ST segment elevation myocardial infarction: executive summary and recommendations. *Circulation* 2001;102:1193–209.

Gibbons R, Chatterjee K, Daley J et al. ACC/AHA/ACP-ASIM Guidelines for the management of patients with chronic stable angina: executive summary and recommendations. *Circulation* 1999;99:2829–48.

Grundy S, Balady GH, Criqui et al. Primary Prevention of Coronary Heart Disease: Guidance from Framingham. *Circulation* 1998;97:1876–87.

Chapter 5

Grundy SM, Pasternak R, Greenland P. Assessment of cardiovascular risk by use of multiple risk factor assessment equations. *Circulation* 1999;100:1481–92.

Klaidman S. *Saving the Heart*. New York, Oxford University Press, 2000.

Myocardial infarction redefined – A consensus document of the Joint European Society of Cardiology/American College of Cardiology Committee for the Redefinition of myocardial infarction. *Eur Heart J* 2000;21:1502–13.

Niebauer J, Dulak J, Chan JR et al. Gene transfer of nitric oxide synthase: effects on endothelial biology. *J Am Coll Cardiol* 1999;34:1201–7

Niebauer J, Hambrecht R, Velich T et al. Attenuated progression of coronary artery disease after 6 years of multifactorial risk intervention: role of physical exercise. *Circulation* 1997;96:2534–41.

Ryan TJ, Antman EM, Brooks NH et al. 1999 update: ACC/AHA guidelines for the management of patients with acute myocardial infarction. A report of the American College of Cardiology/American Heart Association Task Force on Practice Guidelines (Committee on Management of Acute Myocardial Infarction). *J Am Coll Cardiol* 1999;34:890–911.

Schuler G, Hambrecht R, Schlierf G et al. Regular physical exercise and low fat diet: effects on progression of coronary artery disease. *Circulation* 1992;86:1–11.

Wood D, De Backer G, Faergeman O et al. Prevention of coronary heart disease in clinical practice. Recommendations of the Second Joint Task Force of European and other Societies on coronary prevention. *Eur Heart J* 1998;19:1434–503.

Wood D, Durrington P, Poulter N et al. Joint British recommendations on prevention of coronary heart disease in clinical practice. *Heart* 1998;80(Suppl. 2):1–29.

Chapter 6

Hypertension

Background

Approximately one in four adults in the western world suffers from hypertension. Of these, 32% are not aware that they have it, 15% are not on any therapy, and 26% are on inadequate therapy. Only 27% are receiving adequate therapy.

Hypertension is a difficult condition to manage because patients are generally asymptomatic and treatment is preventative rather than palliative. Convincing patients of the need for poorly tolerated medication in the face of well-being is one of the challenges confronting clinicians involved in improving the cardiovascular morbidity and mortality caused by high blood pressure (BP). If untreated, hypertension has serious consequences, including renal disease, myocardial infarction (MI), and cerebrovascular accident. However, many patients do not receive sufficiently aggressive management.

Definition

There is no natural cut-off between normal and high BP. As a result, many threshold values for treatment have been proposed. **Table 1** provides a synthesis of guidelines from the major bodies. Accurate BP measurements are complicated by several factors. For example, there is an approximately 12/7 mm Hg difference between BP measurements taken in the clinic and those taken at home – and in many patients it can be significantly more. Similarly, measurements in the clinic cannot control for a large element of random biological variation, diurnal

	Clinic measurement (mm Hg)	Home measurement (mm Hg)
Optimal control	<140/85	<130/80
Mild hypertension	140–150/90–100	135–145/85–95
Moderate hypertension	150–170/100–110	145–165/95–105
Severe hypertension	>170/110	>165/105

Table 1. Guidelines for threshold values between normal and high blood pressure.

variation, and variation due to chance stress (eg, stress due to being in a traffic jam on the way to the clinic). Consequently, it is recommended that at least three readings are taken.

The annual risk of death from cardiovascular disease (including stroke) or coronary artery disease can be calculated from the European Society of Cardiology tables or Framingham risk tables. Some bodies recommend that mild hypertensives should only be treated if their cardiovascular risk exceeds 2% per year. This consideration of individual risk is welcome, since until recently most clinical trials have involved head-to-head comparisons of monotherapy, whereas in practice most patients require combination therapy.

Causes

No cause is identified in 95% of hypertension patients. However, awareness of treatable causes is important, especially in younger patients in whom there is a higher probability of the hypertension being secondary to some other cause. Causes of secondary hypertension are outlined in **Table 2**.

Assessment

History

History-taking is straightforward since, in most cases, hypertension is asymptomatic. However, symptoms can include headaches, transient ischemic attacks, mild visual disturbances, epistaxes, exertional dyspnea (if heart failure has developed), angina, claudication, weight gain (in Cushing's syndrome), nocturia, and hematuria (with renal disease).

A full drug history is important and must include pharmacologically active preparations such as the combined contraceptive pill and herbal remedies, which are often not regarded by patients as drugs. Other important medications are steroids, sympathomimetics (eg, in cold cures), and nonsteroidal anti-inflammatory drugs, which can reduce the antihypertensive effect of angiotensin-converting enzyme inhibitors (ACEIs) and β-blockers.

As with any cardiovascular disease, risk factors should be especially well documented. As full a family tree as possible should be drawn to document hypertension, diabetes, or early cardiac death. A history of smoking and physical activity should also be taken. More specific to hypertension, caffeine and alcohol intake should be recorded and some insight into diet and lifestyle stress should be acquired.

Hypertension

Causes of secondary hypertension
Renal
• Renal artery stenosis
• Polycystic kidney disease
• Chronic reflux nephropathy
• Chronic glomerulonephritis
• Polyarteritis nodosa
• Systemic sclerosis
Endocrine
• Cushing's syndrome
• Conn's syndrome
• Pheochromocytoma
• Acromegaly
• Hyperparathyroidism
• Polycystic ovarian syndrome
• Metabolic syndrome (diabetes mellitus, dyslipidemia, obesity)
Other
• Obstructive sleep apnea
• Aortic coarctation
• Pre-eclampsia
• Drugs (combined oral contraceptive pill, cyclosporin, steroids)
• CNS disturbances (raised intracranial pressure, familial dysautonomia)

Table 2. Causes of secondary hypertension. CNS: central nervous system.

Examination

The physical examination has three specific objectives:

- documenting an accurate BP
- excluding possible secondary causes
- quantifying end-organ damage

The BP should be measured in both arms, with the arm and manometer at the patient's heart level. Readings should be taken manually in a standardized way (most clinical trials use Korotkoff I and V – from the first sound heard to the complete disappearance of sounds). The use of a large-diameter cuff is essential in those with large arms.

The general appearance of the patient may suggest Cushing's syndrome, a thyroid disorder, polycystic ovarian disease, sleep apnea, or acromegaly. All peripheral pulses should be taken to screen for vascular disease, but special attention should be paid, especially in young people, to radiofemoral delay (diminished and late pulses in the femoral arteries), which suggests aortic coarctation. If positive, the BP should be measured in all four limbs. Auscultation should also be carried out over the aorta and renal arteries for bruits suggestive of stenosis. Abdominal examination may reveal palpable kidneys in polycystic disease or a pheochromocytoma.

End-organ damage can be detected by palpation of the apex beat, detection of bibasal crackles, and examination of the fundi. Diagnosis of hypertensive retinopathy is based on a four-stage grading system, as outlined in **Table 3**.

Investigations

Investigations are aimed at diagnosing rare secondary causes and quantifying end-organ damage.

Only electrolytes, creatinine, fasting glucose, and lipids should be requested in every patient. A low potassium and raised sodium level suggests hyperaldosteronism – either primary (Conn's syndrome) or secondary to renal artery stenosis. This should prompt measurement of renin and aldosterone levels. It should be noted that the potassium level is normal in 50% of cases of primary hyperaldosteronism.

Raised calcium levels suggest possible hyperparathyroidism. If the symptoms suggest a thyroid problem, thyroid function should be tested. A low threshold should be adopted for the following:

- renal ultrasound
- urine microscopy (for casts and cells – glomerulonephritis)
- urine samples for testing:
  - catecholamine metabolites (three samples, one every 24 hours, required in acid bottles)
  - urinary free cortisol (one sample in a plain bottle – this can also be used for glomerular filtration rate and 24-hour protein tests)

Once hypertension has caused end-organ damage, the risks associated with any given level of BP are higher. Evidence of end-organ damage should therefore be sought in all patients. Dip-stick urinalysis, tests for urea and electrolytes, and a renal ultrasound can reveal renal insufficiency. Left ventricular hypertrophy (LVH) can be readily detected by electrocardiography or echocardiography (a chest x-ray

Stage	Signs
I	Arteriolar narrowing and tortuosity
	Increased light reflex
	"Silver wiring"
II	Arteriovenous nipping
III	Cotton-wool "exudates"
	Flame and blot hemorrhages
IV	Papilledema

Table 3. Stages of hypertensive retinopathy (Keith–Wagener classification).

is rarely necessary). Hypertension with LVH carries a particularly poor prognosis (the 5-year mortality is around 30%–40%) and is a powerful predictor of cardiovascular and all-cause mortality.

A useful tool, both for generalists and specialists, is the 24-hour ambulatory BP recording. It is particularly useful when clinic measurements show variability, with resistant hypertension, or most commonly to diagnose "white coat" hypertension. An ambulatory BP measurement (ABPM) is not required for those who are at high risk already, either because of target organ damage or cardiovascular complications. Such patients can be treated on the basis of clinic measurements. Equally, an evidence-based approach suggests that those with mild hypertension, no target organ damage, and low estimated risk may be left untreated (but followed) without ABPM.

Management

Many randomized controlled trials have shown that BP reduction prevents the complications of hypertension. Early trials showed a significant improvement in the risk of stroke, but little or no reduction in coronary heart disease (CHD) events. Later trials, particularly those in the elderly, have also shown a reduction in CHD events, although the benefit is not as great as observational studies predicted. A summary of hypertensive treatments is shown in **Table 4**.

Lifestyle change

Lifestyle changes are important in the management of patients with hypertension and can be used alone during an initial period for those with mild hypertension and low risk.

Chapter 6

Measure	Relative risk↓	Organ protection	Prognosis/ improvement
Lifestyle change	+	+/–	+
Diuretic	+	+	+
Beta-blocker	+	+	+
ACE inhibitor	+	+	+
Ca^{2+} antagonist	+	+	+/–
Angiotensin receptor blocker	+	+	–
Alpha-blocker	+	+/–	–

Table 4. Summary of hypertensive treatment. ACE: angiotensin-converting enzyme. +/–: effect is unclear.

Increasing fruit and vegetable intake can improve BP via an effect on potassium; in combination with a low-fat diet, this can reduce BP by up to 11/6 mm Hg. In addition, weight loss is associated with an approximately 2.5/1.5 mm Hg drop for each kilogram lost. Specific advice on abstaining from adding salt to food – during cooking and at the table – should be given to reduce salt intake to 1 teaspoon per day. Foods such as bread, stock cubes, and breakfast cereals are often surprisingly high in salt. Reducing salt intake can cut BP by approximately 5/3 mm Hg. Alcohol, particularly when taken in a binge pattern, is associated with increased risk. The current American Heart Association guidelines state: "If an individual chooses to consume alcohol, the limit should be one drink [ie, half a pint of beer, one glass of wine, or one short drink] a day for women and two drinks a day for men. People who do not normally drink alcohol should not begin drinking." Regular exercise (walking rather than weight training), stopping smoking, and limiting caffeine intake can all assist in lowering BP and may independently reduce cardiac risk.

Pharmacotherapy

In most patients, altering lifestyle factors is not enough. For these people, there is the difficult balance of pharmacotherapy. Fewer than half of all hypertensive patients can be controlled on monotherapy, whilst one third require three or more drugs. Knowledge of the mechanisms of action of antihypertensives is important as it allows rational combinations to be chosen based on complementary mechanisms of action.

There are four major groups of drug treatments for hypertension and several less frequently used classes. The sites of action of these antihypertensive agents are shown in **Figure 1**.

Hypertension

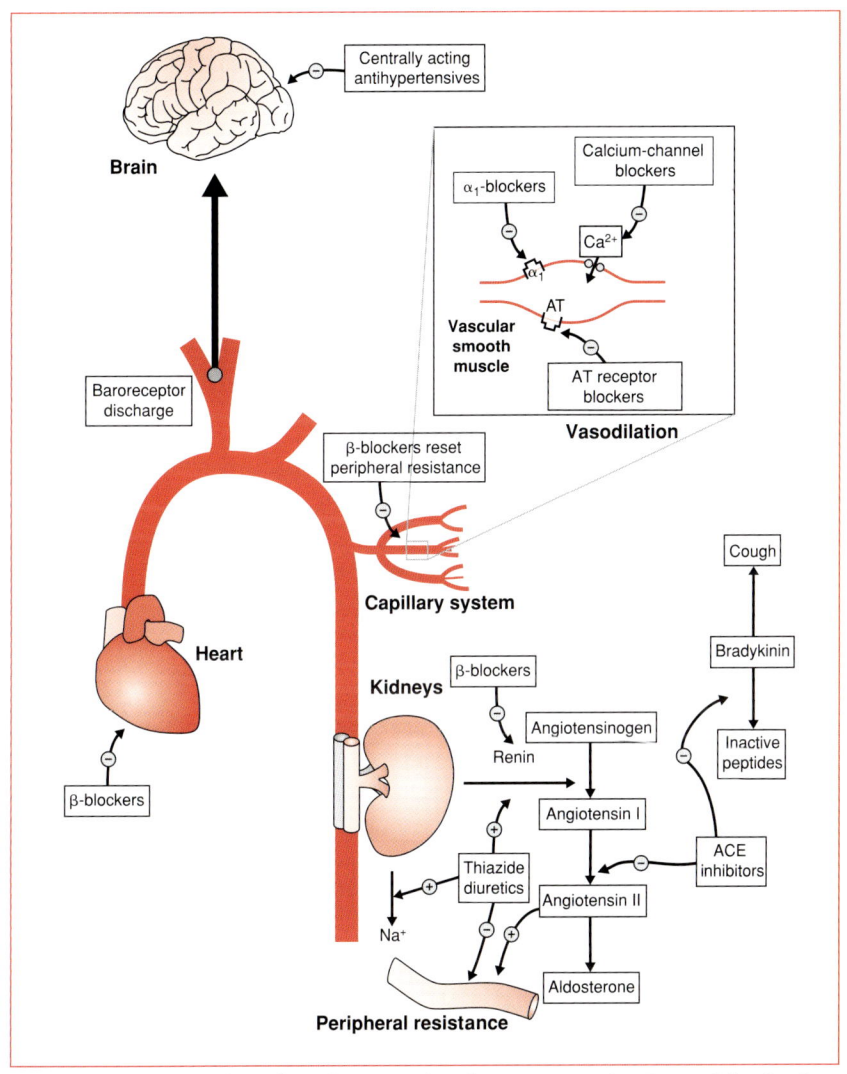

Figure 1. Major physiological mechanisms of antihypertensives. See **Figure 2** for details of centrally acting hypertensives. ACE: angiotensin-converting enzyme; AT: angiotensin.

Beta-blockers

Beta-adrenoreceptor blockers have been used for many decades in the treatment of hypertension and are one of the few classes of agents that have been proven to reduce mortality. They work by reducing cardiac output via negative inotropic and chronotropic actions. In addition, they block sympathetic nervous system stimulation of renin release by juxtaglomerular cells. As with all medications, their

83

use is limited primarily by adverse effects. Asthma is generally considered to be an absolute contraindication, even with agents selective for the cardiovascular system (β_1-receptors). Peripheral vascular disease and bradycardia are relative contraindications. In susceptible patients, heart block and heart failure may be initiated.

The most commonly reported adverse effect is lethargy, and nightmares can occur with lipid-soluble β-blockers. As with all antihypertensives, erectile dysfunction (ED) is a problem. The best guide as to whether ED is iatrogenic is to determine whether the symptoms appeared suddenly. Nevertheless, β-blockers have significant advantages in patients with coexistent angina and anxiety, and also after MI.

Diuretics
Thiazide diuretics, such as bendrofluazide, are another class of agent for which randomized controlled trial evidence indicates an improvement in survival, and should be the first-line drug in the elderly and in those with systolic hypertension. They work by inhibiting NaCl reabsorption in the distal tubule. This initially leads to an increase in Na^+ loss and a reduction in plasma volume. However, the plasma volume soon recovers, leaving a reduced total peripheral resistance, for which the mechanism is unknown. Thiazide diuretics are widely used and very cheap, with a moderate side-effect profile (most commonly hypokalemia, dyslipidemia, and gout). Potassium levels should be checked regularly.

Loop diuretics have a role to play in the place of thiazides when renal function is compromised (creatinine >180 μmol/L or 2 mg/dL) and on a short-term basis, in addition to thiazides, in resistant hypertension, where a significant proportion of patients suffer plasma volume overload.

Calcium-channel blockers
A large number of calcium-channel blockers have been developed and there is good evidence of their ability to reduce BP. There are three subclasses: the dihydropyridines (nifedipine-like), the phenylalkylamine derivatives (verapamil), and the benzothiazepines (diltiazem). All work by blocking the entry of calcium into the smooth muscle cells of resistance vessels, thereby causing vasodilatation. Dihydropyridines cause vasodilatation without the bradycardic and negatively inotropic effects of diltiazem and verapamil (which limits the use of the latter agents to patients with normal left ventricular function) – so a simpler classification is "rate-limiting" and "non-rate-limiting". Short-acting dihydropyridines have become unpopular following reports of increased risk of MI at high doses. Longer-acting calcium-channel blockers are useful antihypertensives, especially as they are lipid-neutral. Side effects include ankle edema, headache, and flushing.

Renin/angiotensin system antagonists

Angiotensin is a potent vasoconstrictor, but also increases activity of the sympathetic nervous system by both central and peripheral mechanisms. Fortunately, the renin–angiotensin system provides a series of targets for pharmacological attack by ACEIs, angiotensin type 1 receptor blockers (ARBs), and aldosterone antagonists (spironolactone). ACEIs and ARBs tend to be well tolerated and have few contraindications, the most important of which is renal artery stenosis. It is important to monitor renal function and potassium levels during initiation and maintenance of these agents. ACEIs are contraindicated in women of child-bearing potential and may cause a troublesome cough through their inhibition of the enzyme responsible for bradykinin degradation. First-dose hypotension can be a problem in elderly patients on diuretics, although newer, longer-acting formulations have reduced this concern. ACEIs are lipid-neutral, improve insulin resistance, and may be able to induce regression of LVH.

Alpha-adrenoceptor antagonists

$Alpha_1$-antagonists (such as doxazosin and prazosin) are becoming more widely used in the treatment of hypertension. They have a good side-effect profile (palpitations and occasional postural hypotension). In addition, they are reported to have beneficial effects on lipid profile and insulin resistance, and lack the negative effects on sexual potency of other antihypertensives, which is a particular advantage for diabetics. They work to reduce total peripheral resistance by blocking the sympathetic activation of α_1-receptors on resistance vessels.

Centrally acting sympathomimetics

Clonidine and α-methyldopa, centrally acting α_2-adrenoceptor agonists, were once popular choices, but are now less widely initiated outside specialist scenarios such as pre-eclampsia. They carry a risk of rebound hypertension on withdrawal.

Other vasodilators

Other vasodilators, such as hydralazine and the very potent minoxidil, are mostly used in resistant hypertension when standard agents fail. Use of the latter is generally restricted by unpleasant side effects such as hypertrichosis.

Imidazoline type 1 receptor agonists

The identification of imidazoline receptors has revealed that the effects of older agents on the central nervous system reflect a relatively nonspecific central site of action mediated primarily through α_2-adrenoceptor agonism (see **Figure 2**). It seems that some of the adverse effects of these agents, which are also mediated through this pathway, can be avoided by the use of selective imidazoline type 1 receptor agents. Early results suggest these agents are well tolerated, with a dry mouth being the only frequently reported unwanted effect (13% at 3 weeks, 2% at 12 months).

Chapter 6

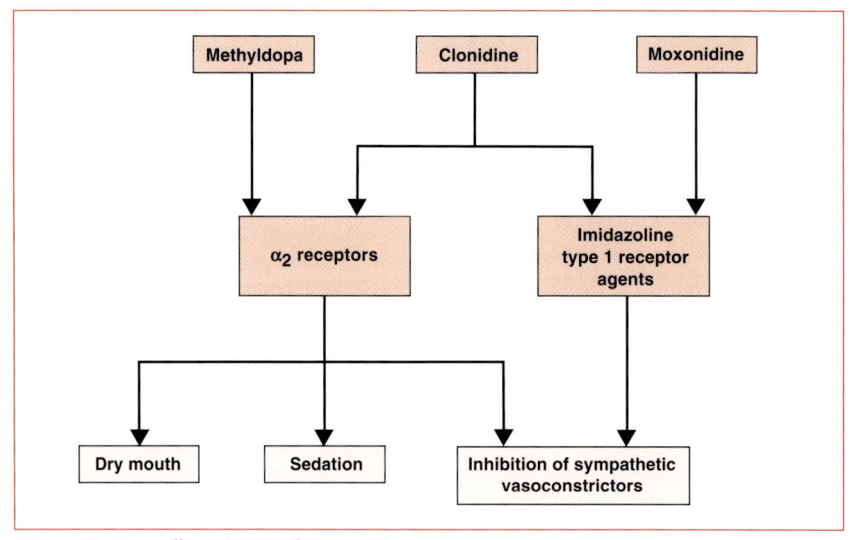

Figure 2. Centrally acting antihypertensives.

Pharmacotherapy selection
In the absence of compelling reasons to choose other medications, the first-line choice should remain a β-blocker or thiazide diuretic. These are the drugs for which clear evidence of mortality reduction exists. In addition, they are generally well tolerated. There are good reasons to consider β-blockers first in younger people and thiazides first in older people. However, the majority of patients will require more than one drug, and the choice should be rational. Here, synergistic action is important (see **Figure 2**). Good combinations are:

- thiazides (which cause secondary hyperreninemia) and ACEIs or ARBs (which block it)
- β-blockers (which act to reduce renin release and cardiac output) and calcium-channel blockers (which cause vasodilatation – do not combine β-blockers with verapamil or diltiazem)

Following this, it is generally worth trying one of the other classes mentioned above. Treatment will be highly individualized depending on patient tolerance and efficacy, but some guidelines are outlined in **Table 5**. It is worth taking readings after each change of drug so that agents with no effect can be stopped.

Systolic versus diastolic hypertension
The question as to the relative importance of systolic and diastolic BP is common in the management of hypertension. For many years it was felt that as systolic hypertension was more common in the elderly it was an inevitable part of aging and arteriolar

	Diuretics	β-blockers	ACE inhibitors
Examples	Bendrofluazide, hydrochlorothiazide	Atenolol, bisoprolol	Lisinopril, ramipril
Particularly good in:	Elderly patients	The young, anxious patients	Diabetics
Contraindicated in:	Gout	Asthma, heart block	Pregnancy, renovascular disease

	Angiotensin type 1 receptor antagonists	Calcium-channel blockers	α-blockers
Examples	Losartan, valsartan	Amlodipine, felodipine	Doxazosin, prazosin
Particularly good in:	ACE cough	Isolated systolic HT	Lipid abnormalities
Contraindicated in:	Pregnancy, renovascular disease	–	Urinary incontinence

Table 5. Guidelines for hypertension pharmacotherapy. ACE: angiotensin-converting enzyme; HT: hypertension.

stiffening. As a result, the focus was primarily on diastolic BP. In fact, both systolic and diastolic BP predict mortality equally well. However, in the elderly population with predominantly systolic BP, recent evidence suggests it is not the absolute values of systolic or diastolic hypertension, but the difference between the two that predicts mortality best, ie, the pulse pressure. This means that a patient with a BP of 160/80 mm Hg may be at higher risk than a patient with a BP of 160/90 mm Hg. This finding, which actually fits well with current thinking on reflected pressure waves in the stiffer arteries of older people, has little therapeutic relevance as yet because we do not have agents that preferentially improve pulse pressure. Thiazides and calcium-channel blockers reduce systolic hypertension more than diastolic, so these are the rational choices. However, the key for the future may be drugs that can restore vascular elasticity, and in this respect nitrates – which donate nitric oxide – are the most promising.

Special populations
Elderly patients
It is a myth that hypertension is "normal" in the elderly and they have less to lose because of a shorter life expectancy. In fact, the absolute benefit from treatment of the elderly is much greater than that for younger hypertensives because of their

larger absolute risk. However, it is true that the prevalence of hypertension is higher amongst the elderly. Optimum BP levels are the same for older people as they are for younger people, and evidence for treatment benefit extends until at least 80 years. Taking pulse pressure into account (see "Systolic versus diastolic hypertension", above), the best agents are thiazide diuretics and long-acting dihydropyridine calcium-channel blockers.

Ethnic groups
Afro-Caribbean blacks have a particularly high prevalence of hypertension and severe complications. Their presentation is unusual in that the renin–angiotensin system is often suppressed. As a result, β-blockers and ACEIs are unlikely to be successful as monotherapy in these patients. Diuretics, calcium-channel blockers, and salt restriction are all effective.

Diabetics
Hypertension is common in diabetics and plays a major role in the vascular complications of the disease. Recent studies have suggested there is more to gain from controlling hypertension in diabetics than there is in achieving normoglycemia. For this reason, particularly aggressive BP-lowering treatment is warranted in these patients. ACEIs, preferably combined with a thiazide diuretic, are the treatment of choice. Previous avoidance of β-blockers or thiazide diuretics because of possible worsening of glycemic control needs to be reassessed in light of this information. Most recent studies show that both groups of drugs can be safely administered in diabetics.

Pregnancy
Hypertension occurs in up to 10% of pregnancies. The key distinction is between chronic hypertension in a pregnant woman and pregnancy-induced hypertension (pre-eclampsia) – defined as a rise in BP of >30/15 mm Hg from early pregnancy. Little is known about which agents are truly safe in pregnancy, but methyldopa is generally considered first line, with calcium antagonists or hydralazine regarded secondarily. Labetalol is sometimes used in the third trimester. In addition, trials in pregnant women with pre-eclampsia have suggested that magnesium sulfate injections may reduce the risk of eclampsia developing by as much as half. ACEIs should be avoided.

Erectile dysfunction
ED is a common problem in hypertensives. It is common because it can be caused by both hypertension (via vascular disease) and its treatment. Differentiating the two from psychogenic causes is a challenge. However, it is made easier by taking a full history: ask about desire, morning erections, erections during masturbation, the exact timing of onset, life stress, sexual history, alcohol, and nonprescription

medication. Palpation of the penis for Peyronie's disease and the testes for atrophy should be added to the routine examination. If ED clearly relates to one particular medication, it is worth trying alternatives. If ED remains resistant, then possible treatments are vacuum devices, intraurethral alprostadil, and sildenafil. Patients with more than three risk factors for coronary disease should have an exercise test before starting sildenafil.

Generalist management

Hypertension is one of the few cardiovascular conditions where, in theory, the generalist can manage the whole process. Because of the overwhelming likelihood that any given hypertensive patient will have "essential" hypertension, only a small number of routine investigations are warranted. These are:

- urine dipstick
- blood glucose, electrolyte, and creatinine levels
- total cholesterol to high-density lipoprotein ratio
- electrocardiography

However, in a young patient, a patient with severe hypertension without a family history, or with signs or symptoms suggesting a secondary cause, the full investigative program detailed above (see "Investigations") should be instituted. This is normally done predominantly within a specialist center.

Refer with confidence

In practice, hypertension specialists tend to see patients from one of the following four categories:

- patients with resistant hypertension
- patients from special groups with hypertension, eg, pregnant women or young people
- patients with known secondary hypertension
- patients with possible accelerated hypertension (see below)

Most generalists would expect to try at least three agents and carry out basic investigations before referring the patient to a specialist for the management of resistant hypertension. Certainly, it would be unusual to make use of vasodilators in the community. However, in the special groups mentioned above, it would not be uncommon for the full work-up to be done from the beginning in a special center. Clearly, any suspicion of accelerated hypertension should result in immediate referral.

Chapter 6

Basic science

BP is a normally distributed, polygenic trait. That is, an individual's BP results from the effects of many genes interacting with each other and the environment. Due in part to this, genetics has so far struggled to explain essential hypertension. However, early studies have suggested that up to 50% of variation within the general population could be explained by genetic factors. The experimental approach has involved studying affected sibling pairs and scanning the whole genome for chromosomal regions with higher levels of genetic marker similarity.

Selectively bred animal models have also been used to study hypertension. Despite much effort, the only mutations that have been convincingly shown to be associated with hypertension are those of the *ACE* gene, and these gene polymorphisms are more strongly associated with atherosclerotic disease than hypertension.

The role of the sympathetic nervous system in hypertension has been debated over many years. Most agree that, together with inadequate salt excretion, it plays an important initiating role (validating the choice of β-blockers as a first-line agent in young hypertensives). However, there is significant controversy as to its continuing role. The prevalent view is that the sympathetic nervous system plays only a minor part in chronic hypertension, and recent studies showing the benefit of ARBs over β-blockers reinforce this.

Resistant hypertension

Failure to reduce BP to <140/90 mm Hg with three or more drugs qualifies the patient as "resistant". Resistant hypertensives commonly suffer plasma volume expansion, despite the absence of clinical signs. In this situation, a more aggressive diuretic therapy can achieve targets where other combinations have failed to do so. Secondary causes are common in resistant hypertensives – they should be referred to a specialist to ensure a full diagnostic work-up. Apparent therapeutic failure could be due to noncompliance; many patients who have been prescribed several different tablets for an asymptomatic condition respond by not taking all of the tablets as directed. Therefore, before altering the medication, determine whether the patient is actually taking it.

Malignant (or accelerated phase) hypertension

In about 1% of patients with hypertension, the condition follows an accelerated course. BP is markedly raised (diastolic >130 mm Hg) and is associated with grade III–IV retinopathy. There may be encephalopathy (headache, confusion, visual disturbance, seizures, and coma), cardiac failure, and rapidly deteriorating renal function. The vascular lesion associated with malignant hypertension is fibrinoid necrosis of the walls of small arteries and arterioles. The prognosis is very poor: untreated, 90% of patients die within 1 year, and even with treatment the 5-year survival rate is only 60%.

Malignant hypertension is a medical emergency that requires immediate therapy. However, the fall in BP should be controlled and carefully monitored as cerebral and myocardial perfusion can become compromised, which could lead to infarction (an initial target diastolic BP should be around 100–110 mm Hg). The reduction in BP is achieved with parenteral agents, such as nitroprusside or labetalol, ideally with intra-arterial BP monitoring. If a pheochromocytoma is suspected, drugs such as phenoxybenzamine or phentolamine (α-adrenergic blockers) should be used first. Once the acute episode has been successfully treated, the BP can be further titrated down over the following weeks.

Further reading

Graves, JW. Management of difficult-to-control hypertension. *Mayo Clin Proc* 2000;75: 278–84.

Hurley ML. New hypertension guidelines. Joint National Committee on Prevention, Detection, Evaluation, and Treatment of High Blood Pressure. *RN* 1998;61:25–8.

Kjeldsen SE, Erdine S, Farsang C et al. 1999 WHO/ISH hypertension guidelines – highlights and ESH update. *J Hypertens* 2002;20:153–5.

O'Brien E, Staessen JA. Critical appraisal of the JNC VI, WHO/ISH and BHS guidelines for essential hypertension. *Expert Opin Pharmacother* 2000;1:675–82.

Ramsay L, Williams B, Johnston G et al. Guidelines for management of hypertension: report of the third working party of the British Hypertension Society. *J Hum Hypertens* 1999;13:569–92.

The American Heart Association guidelines are available at http://www.americanheart.org.

European guidelines are available at http://www.escardio.org.

Chapter 7

Heart failure

Background

The survival rate for myocardial infarction (MI) has greatly increased in recent years due to the success of thrombolysis and primary angioplasty. However, the ensuing epidemic of heart failure has created a major public health problem. Data from the UK suggest that heart failure affects approximately 2% of the population. Furthermore, the prognosis for chronic heart failure (CHF) is poor: a patient admitted to hospital with pulmonary edema has a poorer prognosis (the 5-year mortality rate is around 50%) than a patient presenting with a carcinoma in any organ other than the lung.

The many causes of heart failure (see **Table 1**) operate through the central mechanism of reduced ventricular function. As a consequence, the heart is unable to perfuse the tissues adequately. The resulting clinical syndrome (see **Table 2**) can be explained by compensatory measures, such as cardiac hypertrophy and activation of the sympathetic nervous system and the renin–angiotensin system.

Heart failure is categorized as either systolic or diastolic. Systolic dysfunction is due to poor left ventricular (LV) contraction, usually expressed as ejection fraction (EF). Heart failure patients with diastolic dysfunction (more common in the elderly) have normal LV ejection fraction; the defect seems to lie in relaxation of the left ventricle and is associated with delayed filling. For the generalist, one clue to diastolic dysfunction lies in the chest x-ray (CXR), which can show signs of congestion without significant LV dilatation. However, echocardiography is required for a firm diagnosis (see Chapter 4, Understanding the echocardiogram).

Causes of heart failure	
Ischemic heart disease	High-output cardiac failure
Aortic or mitral regurgitation (volume stress)	Anemia
Aortic or mitral stenosis (pressure stress)	Thyrotoxicosis
Congenital cardiomyopathy	Septicemia
Constrictive pericarditis	Paget's disease
Alcohol excess	Acromegaly

Table 1. Causes of heart failure.

Chapter 7

System	Change
Heart	Left ventricular hypertrophy
	Left ventricular dilatation
	Changes in calcium-cycling proteins
	Switch to fetal isoforms of contractile proteins
	Atrial natriuretic peptide release
	Brain natriuretic peptide release
	Release of proinflammatory cytokines (eg, TNF)
Lungs	Excessive ventilation
	Increased dead space
Kidneys	Renin release
	Erythropoietin release
	Decrease in glomerular filtration rate
	Sodium and water retention
Posterior pituitary	Antidiuretic hormone (vasopressin) release
Adrenal glands	Aldosterone increase
	Catecholamine release
Autonomic nervous system	Activation of sympathetic system
Arteries	Vasoconstriction
	Endothelin release
Skeletal muscles	Endothelial dysfunction
	Changes to metabolism
	Wasting
	Release of proinflammatory cytokines (eg, TNF)

Table 2. The multiorgan symptoms of heart failure. TNF: tumor necrosis factor.

Pathophysiology

The approach to heart failure has changed enormously over the past few years (see **Figure 1**). Earlier thinking focused on inadequate pump function and the accepted therapeutic wisdom was to bolster it with β-agonist inotropes. The idea of treating heart failure by blocking the sympathetic nervous system would have been regarded as heretical and dangerous. However, it has now been realized that most CHF pathology is a result of the body's own compensatory mechanisms (see **Figure 2**) and that interrupting these neurohumoral pathways achieves more than attempting to "overdrive" the failing heart. The exception is acute decompensation (acute heart failure, pulmonary edema, cardiogenic shock), where the focus is on short-term survival; although the primary aim is still the reduction of preload and

(a) The old treatment paradigm

↓ Pump function → Underperfusion of organs → Fluid overload

Treatment: ↑ Pump function using β-agonists

(b) The new treatment paradigm

↓ Pump function → Underperfusion of organs → ↑ ADH, ↑ Renin–angiotensin system, ↑ Sympathetic system

Renin–angiotensin system → Vasoconstriction → ↑ Afterload

↑ ADH → Volume overload → ↑ Preload

↑ Sympathetic system → Tachycardia → ↓ Coronary perfusion

Frank–Starling curve (Force vs End diastolic pressure)

Treatment: interrupt neurohormonal pathways

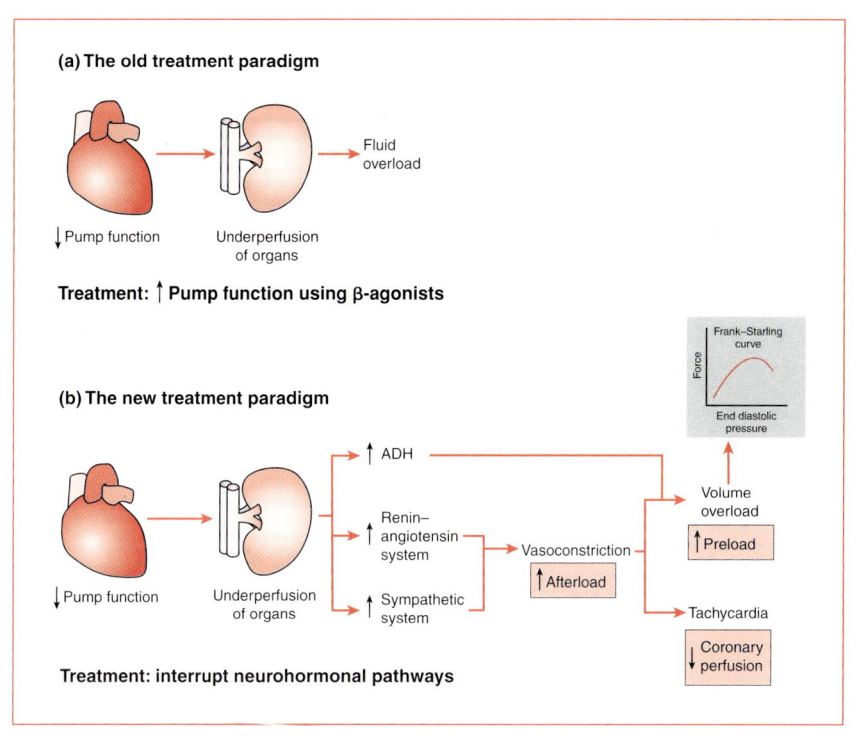

Figure 1. Treatment of heart failure according to (**a**) old and (**b**) new paradigms. ADH: antidiuretic hormone (vasopressin).

afterload using diuretics and vasodilators, inotropes in the form of β-agonists are also used.

Clinical history and examination

The hallmark of heart failure is dyspnea. The classic combination of raised jugular venous pressure (JVP), peripheral edema, palpable liver, basal crepitations, tachycardia, and a third heart sound is well known. Orthopnea (shortness of breath when lying flat) and paroxysmal nocturnal dyspnea (acute nocturnal shortness of breath) are both manifestations of decompensation of ventricular function – precipitated by diurnal susceptibility and increased venous return resulting from adoption of the supine position.

In an elderly person, the cause of acute shortness of breath can often be difficult to diagnose, and the chest may reveal nothing but coarse breath sounds throughout. In this situation, two factors are helpful: the JVP and overt sympathetic overactivation (cold peripheries and profuse sweating).

Chapter 7

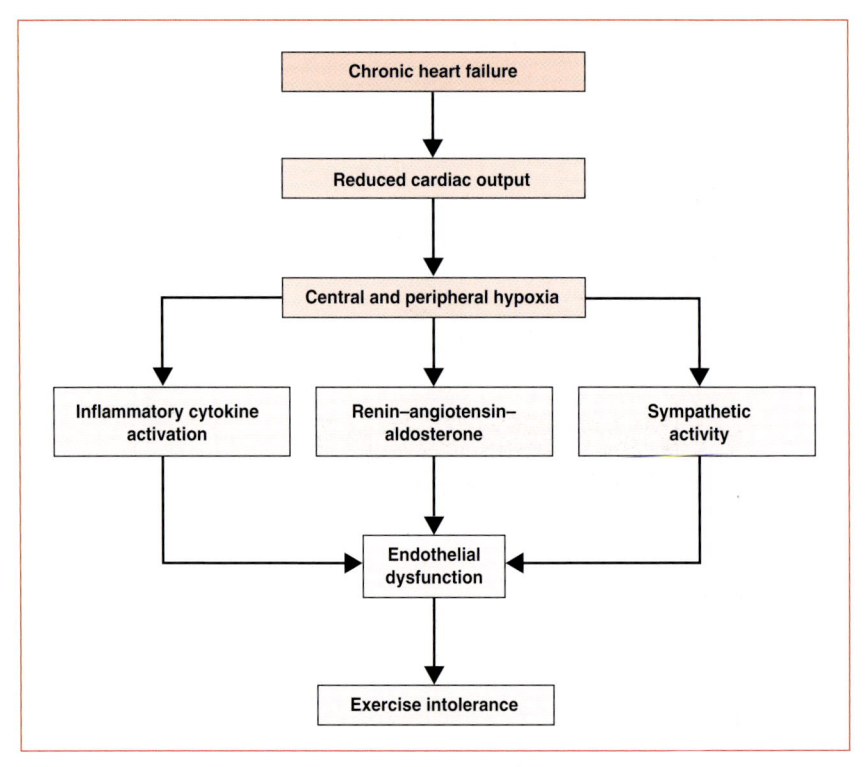

Figure 2. Chronic heart failure. TNF: tumor necrosis factor.

Investigations

Electrocardiography
The electrocardiogram of a patient with heart failure often shows LV hypertrophy (LVH). This may show a "strain" pattern (LVH plus ST depression), most commonly in the lateral chest leads. Arrhythmias are also common in heart failure.

Chest x-ray
Classic signs on CXRs are common only for acute heart failure. Typically, some of the following signs are seen (see **Figure 3**):

- cardiomegaly (see **Figure 4**)
- upper lobe blood diversion
- "bat's wing" alveolar edema
- pleural effusions
- Kerley B lines (lymphatics)

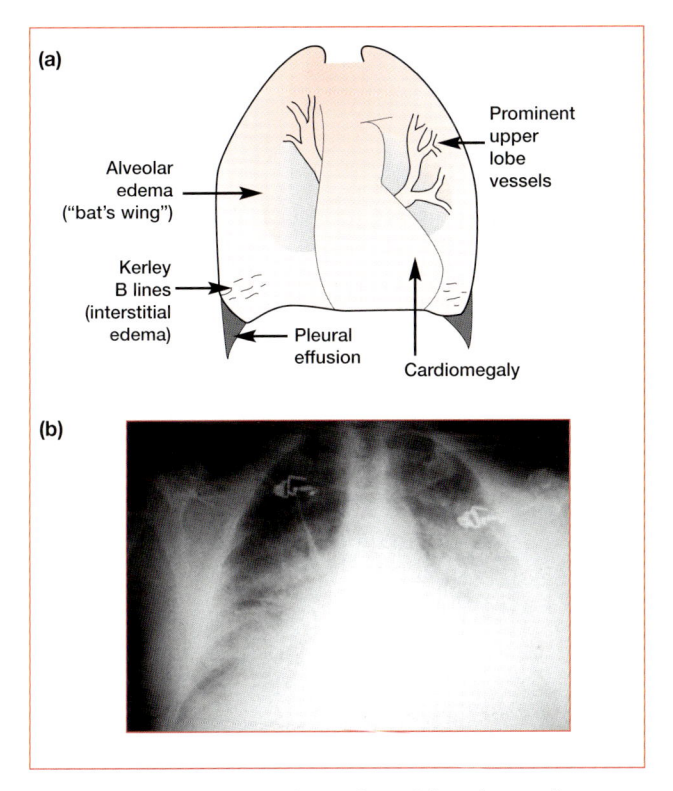

Figure 3. (a) Classic signs of acute heart failure that can be seen on a chest x-ray of left ventricular failure. (b) Pleural effusion on a chest x-ray.

Echocardiography
This is the investigation of choice and can identify and quantify LVH and dysfunction (both systolic and diastolic) as well as examine causes of heart failure, such as valve abnormalities.

Blood tests
The measurement of natriuretic peptides for the diagnosis of heart failure is not yet routine. However, other blood tests can contribute to the clinical picture. The sodium concentration is often low (<130 mmol/L, despite high total body sodium) as a result of dilution and is a strong prognostic indicator. The potassium level is altered by many of the therapeutic agents and should be kept in the mid to high normal range (4.25–5 mmol/L) to minimize the risk of arrhythmia. If the pulse is of full volume, investigative blood tests for anemia and thyroid function should be carried out. If echo suggests restrictive cardiomyopathy, further tests can be carried out for iron storage disease, amyloidosis, or sarcoidosis.

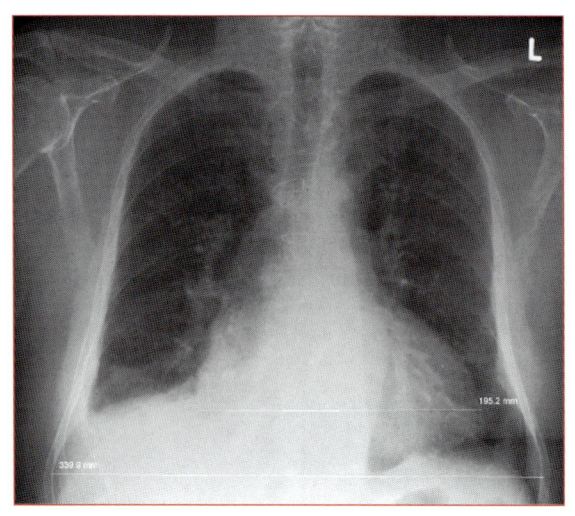

Figure 4. Cardiomegaly and pleural effusion (on the right side) in a patient with heart failure.

Management: acute heart failure

The approach to the management of acute decompensation is different from that to CHF. Acute pulmonary edema should be managed by:

- sitting the patient up
- giving high-flow oxygen
- giving diamorphine (2.5–5 mg intravenous [IV])
- giving nitrates (sublingual at first, then isosorbide mononitrate 2–10 mg/hour IV)
- giving loop diuretics (eg, furosemide [frusemide] 40–80 mg slow IV)

Blood pressure is a key measurement and should be considered when deciding the rate of a nitrate infusion or whether to use β-agonists. If the systolic blood pressure drops below 100 mm Hg, consideration should be given to replacing the nitrate infusion with one containing dobutamine (2–10 μg/kg/min). Although the effect of an IV diuretic can often be dramatic (probably due to an early effect on pulmonary venous dilatation), nitrates are preferred because, in addition to decreasing preload, they also decrease peripheral resistance and do not reduce cardiac output.

It is also important to take the precipitating factor into account. If, for example, a patient is in atrial fibrillation, slowing the ventricular rate may be more effective than a combination of more general measures. Similarly, if a patient has suffered an MI then thrombolysis or intervention may be the key to their recovery.

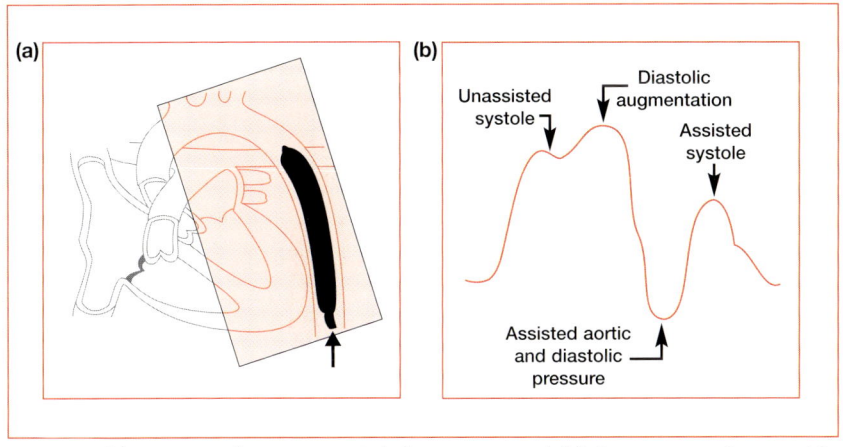

Figure 5. (a) Insertion of an intra-aortic balloon pump and (b) the corresponding arterial pressure waveform.

Management: cardiogenic shock

Cardiogenic shock, which has a 90% mortality rate, is the most severe form of acute heart failure. It is diagnosed when acute heart failure and hypotension are resistant to the measures described above and there is evidence of tissue hypoxia. Treatment, which should be in the coronary care unit of a specialist center, involves inotropic support, invasive monitoring equipment, intra-aortic balloon pumping, and, in the setting of MI, cardiac catheterization.

Intra-aortic balloon pump counterpulsation

Intra-aortic balloon pump (IABP) counterpulsation was developed in the early 1960s. A balloon is inserted, via the femoral artery, into the descending aorta (see **Figure 5**). Using electrocardiography for synchronization, the balloon is almost instantaneously, automatically inflated with helium at the onset of diastole, then deflated just prior to systole. This serves a dual purpose:

- it improves coronary blood flow by increasing the perfusion pressure in the ascending aorta during diastole
- it encourages systemic perfusion by reducing impedance to ventricular ejection at the point of balloon deflation (it creates a negative pressure which helps to "suck" the blood out)

Contraindications to IABP include severe aortic regurgitation and aortic dissection.

Class	Classification
I	No limitation of physical activity. No shortness of breath, fatigue, or heart palpitations with ordinary physical activity.
II	Slight limitation of physical activity. Shortness of breath, fatigue, or heart palpitations with ordinary physical activity, but patients are comfortable at rest.
III	Marked limitation of activity. Shortness of breath, fatigue, or heart palpitations with less than ordinary physical activity, but patients are comfortable at rest.
IV	Severe to complete limitation of activity. Shortness of breath, fatigue, or heart palpitations with any physical exertion and symptoms appear even at rest.

Table 3. The New York Heart Association functional classification of chronic heart failure.

Management: chronic heart failure

The chronic form of heart failure is a condition that most generalists treat every day. When referring these patients, it is useful to classify the severity of heart failure. This is facilitated by a very simple scale: the New York Heart Association (NYHA) functional classification (see **Table 3**). It is straightforward and provides a common language that is understood by cardiologists worldwide.

Diagnosis and assessment

The initial diagnosis and assessment of the severity and progression of CHF can be made using echo and exercise testing with gas analysis. The most commonly used echo measure is the EF. This is rated as:

- 45%–70%, normal
- 35%–45%, mildly impaired
- 25%–35%, moderately impaired
- <25%, severely impaired
- <15%, end-stage/transplant candidates
- 5% is compatible with life, but not long life

The single best exercise-testing measurement is the maximum rate of oxygen consumption (VO_2 max). In a situation where cardiac and respiratory causes of dyspnea coexist, exercise testing with gas analysis can be particularly useful in discerning which is the greater problem.

Treatment

The first step in the management of CHF is patient education. It is easy for physicians to forget (since they use the term every day) that, to most patients, heart "failure"

> **HISTORICAL HEARTS**
> Hippocrates believed that the left side of the heart and its associated arteries were conduits for air rather than blood. Galen (AD 138–201) thought that blood passed through invisible pores in the ventricular septum. Such was his influence on Roman medical thinking that this idea remained in place until the 15th century when an embargo on the dissection of human cadavers was lifted by the Pope. Not long after this, Leonardo da Vinci and others began to produce detailed anatomical drawings, and William Harvey finally described the function of the heart as a pump that pushed blood through a circulatory system, beat by beat.

sounds significantly worse than "myocardial infarction", "heart attack", or even "cardiac arrest". Educating patients about their condition – by giving them information about avoiding excessive salt intake and teaching them how to use their daily weight to monitor fluid balance – will pay dividends in long-term management.

Spironolactone, angiotensin-converting enzyme inhibitors (ACEIs), and β-blockers are the only agents that have been shown to reduce heart failure mortality, and all are now widely used in the community. However, their use requires caution. Although not strictly necessary, most practitioners use short-acting preparations (eg, captopril, metoprolol) when first starting these treatments.

Diuretics
Although diuretics are the mainstay of CHF management, their main role is in symptom control – they may even increase neurohumoral activation. An approach that allows patients to take control of their own diuretic dosage and alter it according to their daily weight (in much the same way as diabetics alter their insulin dosage) may be successful in many patients. It is recommended that diuretics should always be used with an ACEI. In addition, the skillful use of diuretics with complementary actions (see **Figure 6**, **Tables 4** and **5**) can aid diuresis and even avoid hospital admission if the balance is upset. Given the choice between increasing the dose of a loop diuretic or adding another agent, it is usually best to add another agent.

Spironolactone has been shown to improve outcomes in stage III–IV heart failure with an effect equivalent to that of ACE inhibition (25 mg spironolactone has a beneficial effect on remodeling, but essentially no effect on potassium levels and diuresis).

Metolazone is a thiazide-like diuretic that has a powerful synergistic action with loop diuretics, so should be used in the community only as a last resort, for short periods, and be accompanied by daily electrolyte checks.

Chapter 7

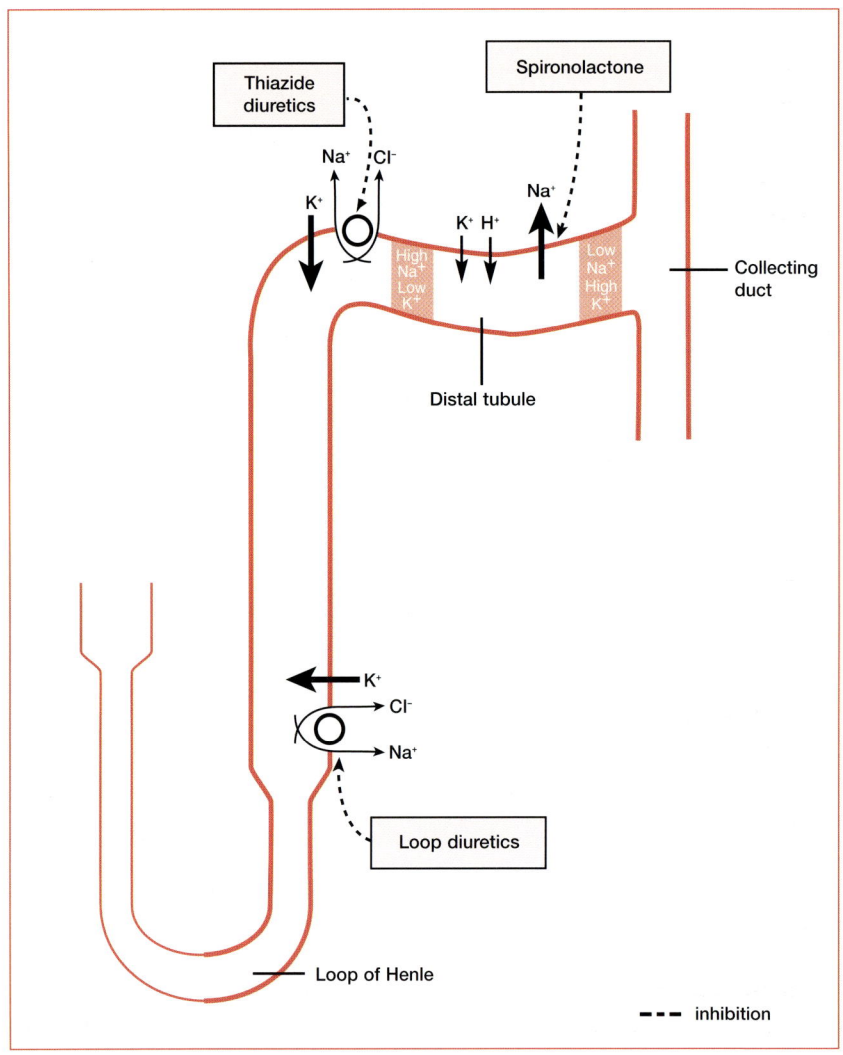

Figure 6. The mechanism of action of diuretics in chronic heart failure management.

> **DEFINING HEARTS**
> *Pulmonary edema was first explained by Henry Welch, who showed that it could be reproduced by obstructing the outflow of the left ventricle. However, the first definition of heart failure was provided by Theophile Bonet (1620–1689), who published clinico-pathological studies linking the effects of valvular disease and cardiac chamber size to the clinical features of dyspnea and edema.*

Class	Compound	Mechanism of action
Loop diuretics	Furosemide (frusemide), bumetanide, torasemide	Inhibit triporter pump in thick ascending loop of Henle, thus inhibiting Na$^+$ and Cl$^-$ reabsorption, which leads to diuresis and potentially hypokalemia
Thiazide diuretics	Bendrofluazide, hydrochlorothiazide	Inhibit NaCl reabsorption in the distal tubule. The greater Na$^+$ load in the distal tubule stimulates Na$^+$ exchange with K$^+$ and H$^+$, causing hypokalemia and metabolic alkalosis
	Metolazone	Particularly potent diuretic, especially when combined with a loop diuretic
Potassium-sparing diuretics	Amiloride	Blocks Na$^+$ channels in the distal nephron
	Spironolactone	Aldosterone antagonist

Table 4. Diuretics used in the treatment of heart failure.

Treatment of heart failure with diuretics

Initial diuretic treatment:
- Loop diuretics or thiazides. Always combine with ACEI
- If GFR ≤30 mL/min do not use thiazides, except as therapy prescribed synergistically with loop diuretics

Insufficient response:
(1) Combine loop diuretics and thiazides
(2) Increase dose of diuretic
(3) With persistent fluid retention – administer loop diuretics twice daily
(4) In severe CHF add metolazone or low-dose spironolactone (25–50 mg) with frequent measurement of creatine and electrolytes

Potassium-sparing diuretics (triamterene, amiloride, spironolactone):
- Use only if hypokalemia persists after initiation of therapy with ACEIs and diuretics
- Start 1-week, low-dose administration
- Potassium supplements are usually ineffective

Table 5. Treatment of heart failure with diuretics (loop diuretics, thiazides, metolazone). ACEI: angiotensin-converting enzyme inhibitor; CHF: chronic heart failure; GFR: glomerular filtration rate. Reprinted with permission from the European Society of Cardiology (Task Force of the Working Group on Heart Failure of the European Society of Cardiology. The treatment of heart failure. *Eur Heart J* 1997;18:736–53).

Chapter 7

> **The recommended procedure for starting an ACEI**
> - Avoid excessive diuresis before treatment. Stop diuretics, if being used, for 24 hours
> - It may be advisable to start treatment in the evening, when supine, to minimize the potential negative effect on blood pressure, although there are no data in heart failure to support this. When initiated in the morning, supervision for several hours with blood pressure control is advisable
> - Start with a low dose and build up to maintenance dosages shown to be effective in large trials
> - Monitor renal function/electrolytes during drug titration every 3–5 days until stable, and then at 3 months and subsequently at 6-monthly intervals. If renal function deteriorates substantially, stop treatment
> - Avoid potassium-sparing diuretics during initiation of therapy. Add potassium-sparing diuretics only with persisting hypokalemia or refractory natriuretic therapy. However, spironolactone can safely be added at a dose of 25 mg, since at this dose it has no effect on potassium levels and diuresis
> - Avoid nonsteroidal anti-inflammatory drugs
> - Check blood pressure 1–2 weeks after each dose increment
>
> The following patients should be referred for specialist care:
> Cause of heart failure unknown
> Systolic blood pressure <100 mm Hg
> Serum creatinine >1.47 mg/dL (130 μmol/L)
> Serum sodium <130 mmol/L
> Moderate or severe heart failure
> Valve disease

Table 6. The recommended procedure for starting an angiotensin-converting enzyme inhibitor (ACEI). Reprinted with permission from the European Society of Cardiology (Task Force of the Working Group on Heart Failure of the European Society of Cardiology. The treatment of heart failure. *Eur Heart J* 1997;18:736–53).

Angiotensin-converting enzyme inhibitors

ACEIs were the first agents shown to reduce mortality in heart failure. Angiotensin receptor blockers (ARBs) are currently reserved for those patients with an ACE cough. Guidelines for starting ACEIs are outlined in **Table 6**.

Beta-blockers

Much of the early work on β-blockers used carvedilol – a nonselective β-blocker, α-antagonist, and antioxidant. However, although its significant effect appeared to result from β-blockade resulting in many different β-blocking agents being used, recent trials have suggested there may be effects over and above that of β-blockade. Beneficial effects of β-blockade include a reduction in heart rate (which increases

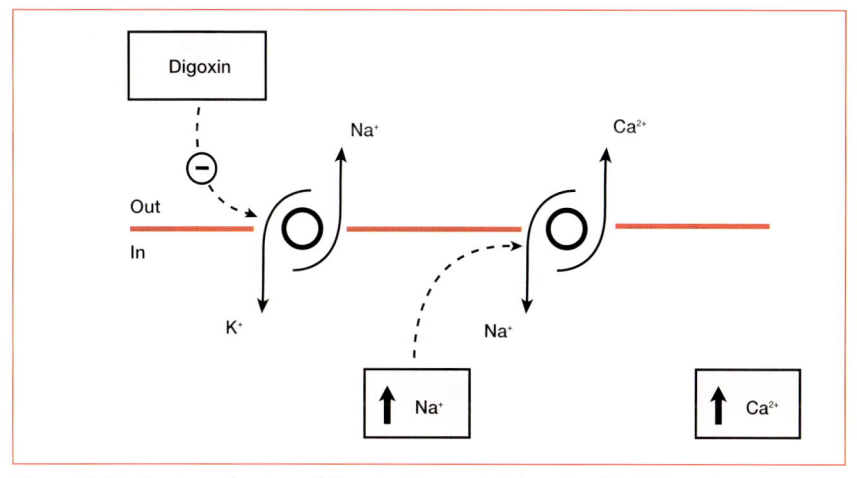

Figure 7. Mechanism of action of digoxin. Digoxin inhibits Na$^+$/K$^+$ ATPase. As a consequence of an increased intercellular Na$^+$ concentration, Ca^{2+} extrusion (via Na$^+$/Ca^{2+} exchange) is reduced. The result is an increase in cellular Ca^{2+}.

myocardial perfusion), regression of LVH (probably related to inhibition of the deleterious effects of excess catecholamines), and a reduction in sudden death (probably related to a reduction in ventricular fibrillation – 50% of heart failure deaths are due to arrhythmia).

Digoxin
Digoxin has perhaps the longest history of any of the treatments for heart failure. However, being a positive inotrope, it occupies a controversial place overarching the old and new paradigms for the treatment of sinus rhythm heart failure. It works by increasing cellular calcium via inhibition of Na$^+$/K$^+$ ATPase and consequent reduction of Ca^{2+} extrusion via Na$^+$/Ca^{2+} exchange (see **Figure 7**). As K$^+$ "competes" with digoxin at the ATPase site, digoxin can become toxic in hypokalemic patients. Symptoms of digoxin toxicity are gastrointestinal upset and (more rarely) visual disturbances and headache. However, despite its widespread use, there have been no large, prospective, placebo-controlled trials to determine the efficacy of digoxin in reducing mortality (although it has been shown to reduce hospital admissions).

Hydralazine and nitrates
The vasodilator combination of hydralazine (up to 300 mg) and nitrates (160 mg isosorbide dinitrate) has been tested with digoxin and diuretics in several large trials and has been associated with mortality reductions in heart failure. However, the advent of ARBs is likely to offer a better alternative to ACEIs than this drug combination.

Chapter 7

NYHA class	Affect outcome						Symptom control only
	ACEI	BB	Spironolactone	ARB	Hydralazine/ nitrates	Digoxin	Diuretic
I	+	+/−	−	−	+	−	+
II	+	+	−	+	+	−	+
III	+	+	+	+	+	+	+
IV	+	+	+	+	+	+	+

Table 7. Treatment of heart failure according to the New York Heart Association (NYHA) functional classification of congestive heart failure. ACEI: angiotensin-converting enzyme inhibitor; ARB: angiotensin receptor blocker; BB: β-blocker.

Future directions

Areas of controversy still exist in the management of CHF. For example, aspirin is known to be effective as an aid to secondary prevention of coronary artery disease. However, it can reduce the efficacy of ACEIs. Also, despite the high rate of heart failure deaths due to arrhythmia (50%), amiodarone is the only antiarrhythmic (so far) that has been shown to reduce mortality.

New agents currently being investigated in trials include:

- calcium sensitizers (increase contractile response to intracellular Ca^{2+})
- endothelin antagonists (there are increased levels of endothelin – a potent vasoconstrictor – in heart failure); results of all recent trials have been negative or neutral at best
- TNF-α antibodies; recent trials all produced negative results
- neutral endopeptidase inhibitors (neutral endopeptidase breaks down atrial natriuretic peptide and brain natriuretic peptide – peptides with diuretic, natriuretic, and vasodilator properties)

Heart failure treatments, according to NYHA classification, are outlined in **Table 7**.

Nonpharmacotherapies

Recent evidence suggests that individualized exercise training programs can be beneficial in stable, mild to moderate heart failure. Like most other aspects of the treatment of heart failure, today's advice (exercise) is the opposite of that from 30 years ago (bed rest).

Heart failure

> **EARLY TREATMENTS**
> *The first breakthrough in the treatment of heart failure was by William Withering (1741–1799), who published observations of the therapeutic use of digitalis (foxglove). Ironically, he believed its main mechanism of action was diuretic. Until the discovery of digitalis, treatment for heart failure had remained unchanged since Egyptian times: bed rest, fluid restriction, and weak herbal diuretics were combined with starvation, laxatives, and venesection. Patients can perhaps derive some solace from the fact they are living today, rather than 200 years ago.*

Revascularization of patients with heart failure is being considered increasingly as it is realized that chronic LV dysfunction does not necessarily mean permanent or irreversible cell damage. Myocardium that has suffered low-level ischemia and no longer contributes significantly to ventricular function (hibernating myocardium) remains viable, and therefore potentially rescuable. It can be detected by cardiovascular magnetic resonance imaging, perfusion imaging, low-dose dobutamine stress echo, or PET scanning (perfusion metabolism mismatch).

Many patients with systolic heart failure exhibit significant intra- or interventricular conduction delays (IVCDs) that cause ventricular dysynchrony, recognized by a wide QRS complex on the ECG (typically, a left bundle branch block morphology). Ventricular dysynchrony has several important consequences for cardiac performance, which include abnormal interventricular septal wall motion, reduced diastolic filling time, and prolonged mitral regurgitation duration. In addition, there is a proportional increase in mortality with increasing QRS duration. Cardiac resynchronization therapy (CRT) provides atrial-synchronized, biventricular pacing using standard pacing technology combined with a special third lead. This third lead is implanted via the coronary sinus and positioned in a cardiac vein to sense and pace the left ventricle. Following a sensed atrial contraction, both ventricles are stimulated to contract simultaneously. The resulting resynchronization of ventricular contraction reduces mitral regurgitation and optimizes left ventricular filling, thereby improving cardiac function.

Transplantation and ventricular assist devices are options for end-stage disease. Local availability and guidelines vary. Indications are:

- severe LV dysfunction (eg, EF <20% as demonstrated by radionuclide ventriculography)
- VO_2 max <14 mL/kg/min (patients with values above this tend to have a better prognosis without surgery)

Contraindications center on comorbidities, eg, vasculopathy, diabetes mellitus with target-organ damage, or pulmonary hypertension. In addition, few centers will transplant patients over the age of 60 years.

Several studies have shown clear benefit from a multidisciplinary approach to heart failure treatment. Specialist nurses who visit patients in the community can significantly reduce the rate of hospitalization by helping with exercise, symptom control, and fluid balance, and by alerting the medical team early to any potential deterioration.

Palliative care

The very poor prognosis associated with heart failure begs the question of the availability of hospice care and end-of-life support for this population. The irony remains that while cancer patients receive end-of-life support and often report dyspnea as an equivalent problem to pain, many more heart failure patients whose chief symptom is dyspnea have a poorer prognosis and go unattended. The management of these patients is an area deserving of more investigation and analysis. For example, what is the place of drugs that are known to help symptoms but which might increase the risk of sudden death (eg, inotropes)? Does "dual-intent" apply? What are the wishes of the patient? As cardiology becomes more technological there is less focus on patients and more on their lesions and the tools used to treat them. Generalists are almost certainly better than cardiologists at practising holistic care.

Unfortunately, conventional drugs for the treatment of heart failure do not adequately control the most common symptoms of fatigue and dyspnea. The latter is the most common distressing symptom in refractory heart failure. Maintaining a very close control of plasma volume is facilitated by regular weighing and adjustment of diuresis, but this rarely provides full symptom control. Fortunately, relief is possible through the use of opiates. These drugs reduce preload and afterload, dampen the central respiratory drive, and relieve distress through a central narcotic action. Thus, they are well suited for use in this situation. Drawbacks, such as tolerance and dependence, should not deter their use as studies suggest that they are minimal in this setting. Physical dependence is inevitable, but only relevant in the case of discontinuation of therapy, in which case it can be managed by gradual withdrawal. Morphine can be given at a dose of 2.5 mg 4 hourly and as required, with the 4-hourly dose readjusted after 48 hours to take account of interim dosing. Control of constipation should always accompany chronic opioid treatment.

Further reading

Jong P, Demers C, McKelvie RS et al. Angiotensin receptor blockers in heart failure: meta-analysis of randomized controlled trials. *J Am Coll Cardiol* 2002;39:463–70.

Krumholz HM, Baker DW, Ashton CM et al. Evaluating quality of care for patients with heart failure. *Circulation* 2000;101:E122–40.

Niebauer J, Volk HD, Kemp M et al. Endotoxin and immune activation in chronic heart failure: a prospective cohort study. *Lancet* 1999;353:1838–42.

Nolan J. A historical review of heart failure. *Scott Med J* 1993;38:53–7.

Task Force of the Working Group on Heart Failure of the European Society of Cardiology. The treatment of heart failure. *Eur Heart J* 1997;18:736–53.

Chapter 8

Arrhythmia

Introduction

Arrhythmia is an area of cardiology often feared by generalists. This might be related to the inconsistent terminology used in different centers and countries; or perhaps because the most basic tool of diagnosis, the electrocardiogram (ECG), can at times seem the most esoteric. Whatever the reason, few feel completely comfortable when confronted with a patient with ongoing arrhythmia. Despite this, arrhythmia can be simply managed by asking the following question: is the patient compromised? This is the first and single most important question in the management of your patient. The answer will guide your next steps.

If the patient is not compromised – no pain, no dyspnea, normal blood pressure, and fully alert – you have some time. Take a short history and examination, get the patient monitored (preferably), and acquire a 12-lead ECG. The findings will help to make a diagnosis that will guide treatment. If a 12-lead ECG is not available, immediately refer the patient to somewhere that it can be performed.

If the patient is compromised – with pain, dyspnea, hypotension, and light headedness – this is an emergency and the patient needs an intravenous (IV) cannula inserted and a defibrillator brought in immediately. Treatment then depends on the diagnosis (see **Table 1**).

Clinical examination can help, whether an ECG is available or not. The key thing to remember is that there are few components in the electrical "wiring" of the heart (see **Figure 1**) and the pulse can only be fast or slow, regular or irregular. If an ECG is available, is the QRS complex narrow or broad? Broad (>0.12 seconds) is more likely to be ventricular tachycardia (VT) and will generally be more concerning than narrow, which suggests a high depolarization site and is likely to be supraventricular tachycardia (SVT).

Bradycardia

Bradycardia is defined as heart rate <60 bpm, regardless of the cause. However, this is not a particularly helpful definition as it is well known that elite athletes can have "normal" heart rates as low as 30 bpm. In general, bradycardia needs

Chapter 8

Pulse	Most likely diagnosis	ECG to rule out
Regular and slow (~60 bpm)	Sinus rhythm Junctional rhythm	Complete heart block
Regular and fast (~150 bpm)	Atrial flutter with 2:1 AV block	Ventricular tachycardia
Regular and fast (>150 bpm)	AV node re-entrant tachycardia	Ventricular tachycardia
Irregular and fast	Atrial fibrillation with rapid ventricular response	Ventricular tachycardia
Irregular and slow	Atrial fibrillation with controlled ventricular response	Ventricular tachycardia

Table 1. Possible diagnoses of an arrhythmic patient. AV: atrioventricular; ECG: electrocardiogram.

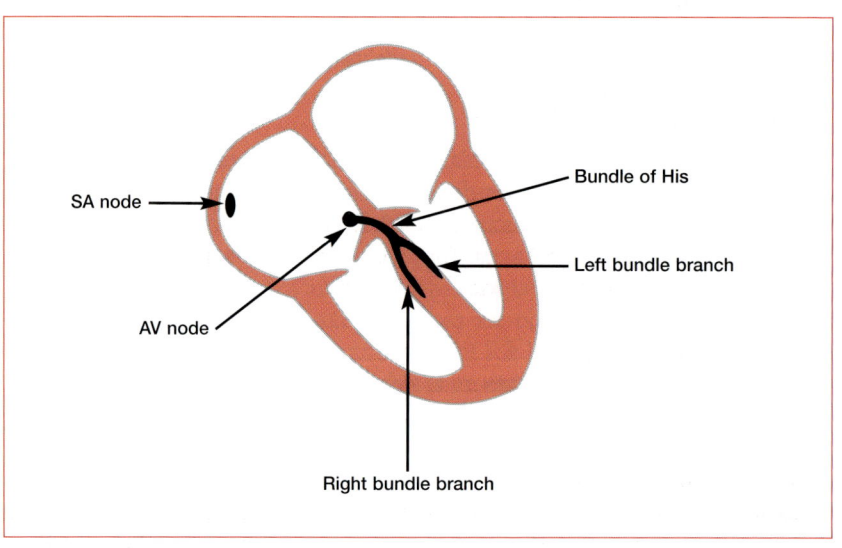

Figure 1. A diagrammatic representation of the electrical "wiring" of the heart. AV: atrioventricular; SA: sinoatrial. Reproduced with permission from Elsevier Science (Hampton J. *The ECG Made Easy*. Churchill Livingstone, 2003).

attention if it is associated with symptoms, hemodynamic compromise, or is the substrate for escape rhythms. Symptoms associated with bradycardia include shortness of breath, fatigue, lethargy, nausea, mental confusion, dizziness, and presyncope or syncope. If there is hemodynamic compromise and interruption of cerebral perfusion is prolonged, *grand mal* seizures may result (Stokes–Adams attacks). The causes of bradycardia are outlined in **Table 2**.

Arrhythmia

Causes of bradycardia	
Physiological	Sinus node disease
• Athletic bradycardia	Atrioventricular node disease
Drugs	Abnormal vagal tone
• Beta-blockers	Carotid sinus hypersensitivity
• Rate-limiting calcium-channel blockers	Malignant vasovagal syndrome
• Digoxin	Raised intracranial pressure
• Amiodarone	Hypothyroidism
Ischemia	Hypothermia

Table 2. Causes of bradycardia.

Treatment

Acute bradycardia only requires treatment if it is associated with hemodynamic compromise or dangerous escape rhythms. This will most often be the case in the setting of inferior myocardial infarction (MI), but check the temperature! IV atropine at a dose of 500 µg can be administered and repeated up to a maximum cumulative dose of 3 mg. If this fails, there are two options.

(1) External pacing. This is a temporizing measure only. Most defibrillators have detachable modules to facilitate this. Attach electrode gels anteriorly and posteriorly and pace at 80 bpm. The procedure is distressing for the conscious patient and should be used with sedative analgesia.

(2) IV isoproterenol (isoprenaline) infusion. If the parasympathetic system is entirely blocked, the only alternative is to stimulate the sympathetic pathway. However, this is proarrhythmic and not without risk.

Sinus node dysfunction

Sinus node dysfunction (SND) is also known as tachycardia–bradycardia syndrome and sick sinus syndrome. These terms encompass a spectrum of disorders of cardiac conduction tissue that are not necessarily confined to the sinus node (eg, atrial conducting tissue and even the atrioventricular [AV] node). The cause is not entirely clear, but inflammation, degeneration, and fibrosis of the conducting tissue are characteristic. SND is most common in the elderly.

The spectrum of associated arrhythmias is diverse, but usually includes inappropriate sinus bradycardia, sinus pauses (>3 seconds) with junctional escape, sinus arrest (asystolic pause), atrial tachycardia, atrial flutter, and atrial fibrillation (AF). Commonly, there is alternating bradycardia–tachycardia with a normal sinus rate or bradycardia between attacks. Hence, the diagnostic landmarks

Chapter 8

are palpitations (tachycardia), dizziness, and syncope (bradycardia), although the disease is often asymptomatic.

SND is diagnosed by a 12-lead ECG and Holter monitoring. Although there is no evidence of mortality benefit (SND does not seem to cause fatal asystolic arrest), consensus exists that a pacemaker (AAI, DDD – see p.135 for a description of the pacemaker codes) should be implanted if there is a clear relationship between bradycardia and cerebral symptoms in the absence of drugs – a diagnosis that may be difficult to secure. In addition, a pacemaker may be considered (AAI, DDD) when bradycardia is secondary to drug therapy necessary to limit tachycardia.

Carotid sinus syndrome

This term refers to hypersensitivity of the baroreceptor reflex, leading to bradycardia and hypotension. It is usually caused when pressure is applied to the neck around the area of the carotid sinus, eg, when shaving or by wearing a tight shirt collar. It can be predominantly cardioinhibitory (bradycardia, AV block) or vasodepressive (hypotension). Diagnosis is by ECG monitoring during carotid sinus massage. Patients with >3 seconds of asystole benefit from permanent dual-chamber pacing (DDI). Single-lead atrial pacing is contraindicated because it offers no protection against AV block. In patients with predominant vasodepressor syncope or mixed forms of the condition, pacing only prevents symptoms due to asystole or bradyarrhythmia; it does not prevent neurologic symptoms due to reflex hypotension.

Syncope

Syncope is defined as a sudden transient loss of consciousness and postural tone with spontaneous recovery. A careful diagnostic evaluation, though often difficult, is imperative in all patients. A vast variety of conditions may result in syncope, including any condition causing relative cerebral hypoxia for ≥10 seconds. It occurs as a result of low cardiac output and can be a consequence of mechanical, rhythm, and vascular disturbances, and noncardiac causes (see **Table 3**).

It should be kept in mind that generalized tonic/clonic movements can be the result of syncope, rather than the cause of it.

Evaluation

It can be difficult to identify the cause of syncope. Initial clinical evaluation should include supine and erect blood pressures and heart rate measurements. Blood glucose, serum electrolytes, hematocrit, and drug levels (if appropriate) should also be obtained. Assessment of a syncopal event requires information from both the patient and a witness; the pattern can be helpful (see **Table 4**). A baseline 12-lead ECG may suggest possible causes such as ischemia, Wolff–Parkinson–White (WPW) syndrome,

Type of disturbance	Examples
Mechanical	Cardiac valvular disease
	Acute myocardial infarction
	Hypertrophic cardiomyopathy
	Tamponade
	Pulmonary embolus
Rhythm	Sinus node dysfunction
	Bradycardia
	Tachycardia
Vascular	Cerebrovascular disorders
	Neurally mediated vasodilatation:
	• malignant vasovagal syndrome
	• carotid sinus syncope
	• drug-induced
Noncardiac causes	Central nervous system substrates, eg, epilepsy, tumor
	Metabolic/endocrine disturbances, eg, hypoglycemia, hyperventilation
	Psychiatric disorders

Table 3. Disturbances that can lead to syncope.

or a prolonged QT interval. In most cases, it will be necessary to refer the patient for additional testing (see **Figure 2**). Additional testing may include the following.

- Documentation of a symptomatic arrhythmia may be achieved by Holter monitoring. However, if syncope is infrequent, event-recorder monitoring may be more helpful. These devices allow patients to turn the device on when the episode begins (or ends, facilitated by the use of a buffer), and thus record over a much greater period of time.
- An echocardiogram should be used to detect major structural abnormalities potentially associated with syncope (aortic stenosis, hypertrophic cardiomyopathy, ischemia). Carotid sinus massage should be performed if bruits are absent.
- Before invasive electrophysiological testing, coronary artery disease should be excluded or treated. Electrophysiological testing is indicated whenever an arrhythmia is considered as a probable cause of syncope.
- Exercise testing may contribute to establishing a basis for syncope by revealing myocardial ischemia (substrate for ventricular tachyarrhythmias), catecholamine-sensitive tachycardias, exercise-induced AV block, and chronotropic incompetence (SND).

	Arrhythmia	Vasovagal	Neurogenic
Premonitory	Often none	Cough, micturition, standing, neck extension	Headache, confusion, aura
Episode	Sudden collapse	Collapse, pale, unconscious <1 minute	Fit, eg, tongue biting, incontinence
Recovery	Feels well	Feels ill	Often prolonged postictal phase

Table 4. Patterns of syncope.

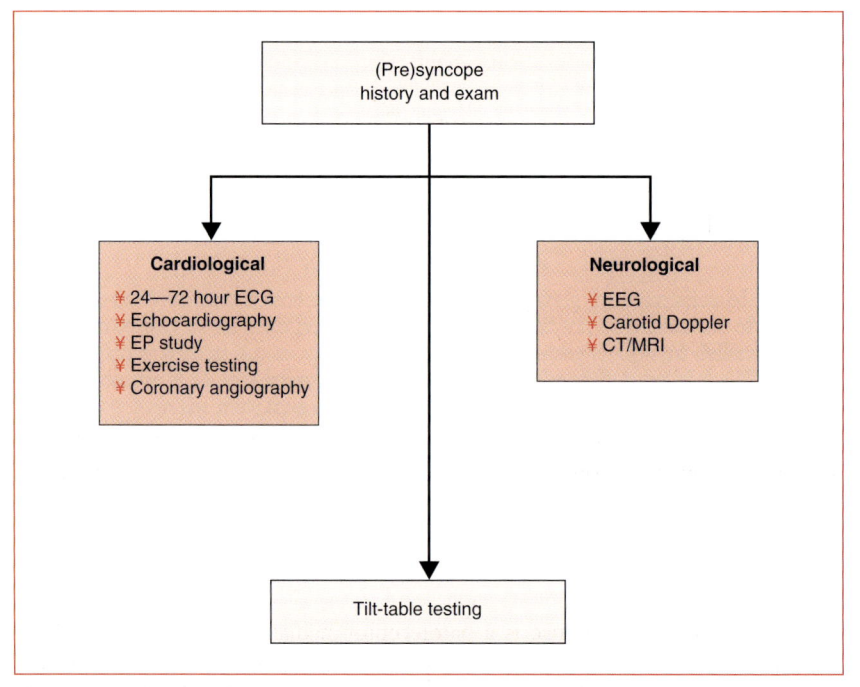

Figure 2. Evaluation of syncope. CT: computed tomography; ECG: electrocardiogram; EEG: electroencephalogram; EP: electrophysiology; MRI: magnetic resonance imaging.

Malignant vasovagal syncope

In malignant vasovagal syncope, the sympathetic system is activated via a trigger, usually venous pooling, which forces vigorous contraction of a poorly filled ventricle. This stimulates the mechanoreceptors in the ventricular wall, which lead (via C fibers and the brainstem) to overactivation of the parasympathetic system, and thus bradycardia and hypotension. This reflex is named Bezold–Jarisch after those who first described it (see **Figure 3**).

Arrhythmia

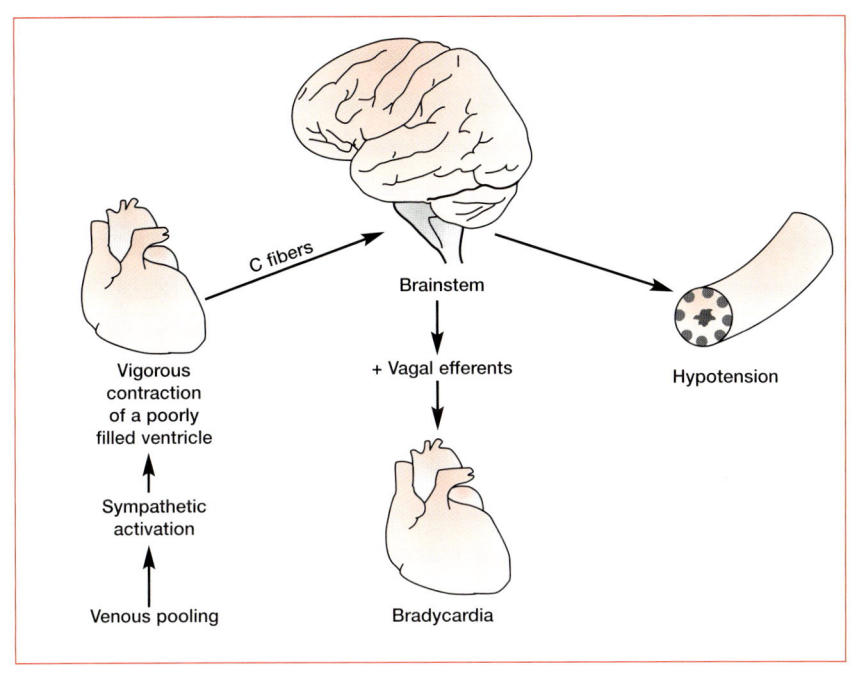

Figure 3. The Bezold–Jarisch reflex.

Tilt-table testing
If malignant vasovagal syncope is suspected, the key investigation is upright tilt-table testing. This test is performed on a specially designed table with the patient initially in a supine position. He/she is then tilted upright to a maximum of 60°–80° in such a way as to avoid recruiting the postural muscles. This maximizes venous pooling. The patient is left in this position for up to 40 minutes.

The normal tilt-table response is a baroreceptor-mediated decrease in inhibitory drive to the vasomotor center, ie, vasoconstriction and an increase in heart rate and ventricular contractility. The test result is considered abnormal when symptomatic hypotension is reproduced (Bezold–Jarisch reflex).

Treatment
Therapy to prevent recurrent vasovagal syncope has included the use of β-blockers and vagolytics (eg, disopyramide).

Atrioventricular block
AV block occurs when the electrical impulse from the atria to the ventricles is delayed or blocked.

First-degree AV block
This is where there is a prolonged PR interval of >200 milliseconds (5 small squares; see **Figure 4**). No specific therapy is required and the prognosis is excellent. However, it can be a marker for an underlying problem such as myocarditis, MI, degenerative disease, or, most commonly, a drug effect (eg, tricyclic antidepressants).

Second-degree AV block
This is divided into two types:

- type I (Mobitz I or Wenckebach AV block)
- type II (Mobitz II AV block)

Type I occurs when there is a repeated pattern of progressive prolongation of the PR interval, which eventually results in the failure of conduction of one atrial beat (see **Figure 5**). The cause is usually benign, but it can be a marker for the same underlying cardiac problems as first-degree AV block. In most cases, treatment is unnecessary. Routine prophylactic permanent pacing is not recommended unless the patient is symptomatic with presyncope, recurrent syncope, or bradycardia that exacerbates congestive heart failure or angina.

In type II, most beats are conducted with a constant PR interval, but occasionally atrial depolarization is not followed by ventricular depolarization (see **Figure 6**). Type II is pathological and indicates disease of the conduction system distal to the AV node. It can frequently lead to complete AV block, causing Stokes–Adams attacks. Therefore, temporary and then permanent pacing (DDD) is indicated in most patients, even those who initially present without symptoms.

Third-degree AV block (complete heart block)
With complete heart block, there is complete dissociation of the P waves and QRS complexes (see **Figure 7**). The ventricular escape complexes are usually wide and occur at around 30–40 bpm. There is a significant risk of asystole and thus permanent pacing (DDD) is indicated, regardless of symptoms. Acquired AV block is most commonly due to ischemic heart disease or drug toxicity (in particular β-blockers, digitalis, and calcium-channel blockers).

Bradyarrhythmia in atrial fibrillation
In patients with intermittent or chronic AF, AV node dysfunction is not an uncommon finding. Clearly, this will be aggravated by many of the rate-limiting drugs given to control the ventricular rate. In these cases, consideration should be given to the implantation of a pacemaker to protect against bradycardia while still allowing pharmacological control of a rapid ventricular rate.

Arrhythmia

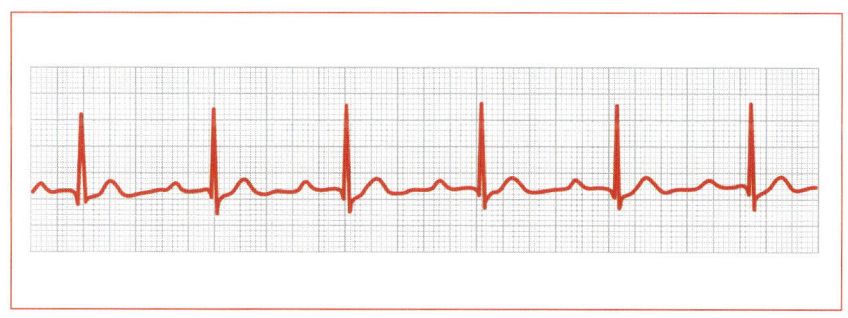

Figure 4. Electrocardiogram of first-degree atrioventricular block.

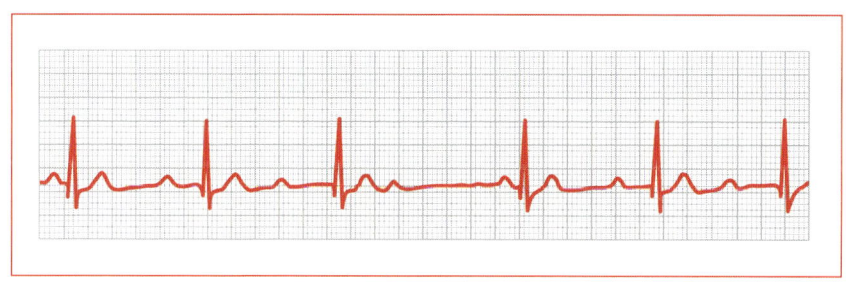

Figure 5. Electrocardiogram of type I second-degree atrioventricular block (Wenckebach).

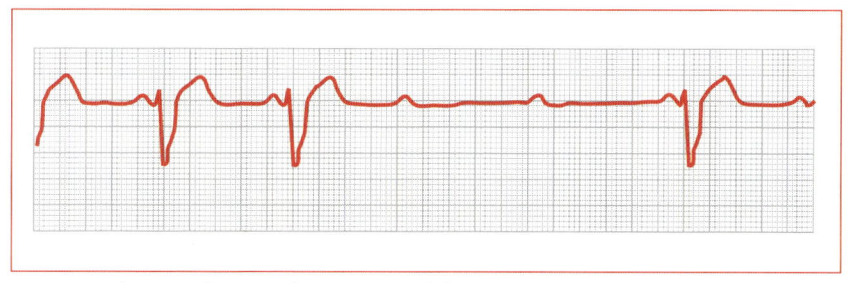

Figure 6. Electrocardiogram of type II second-degree atrioventricular block (Mobitz II).

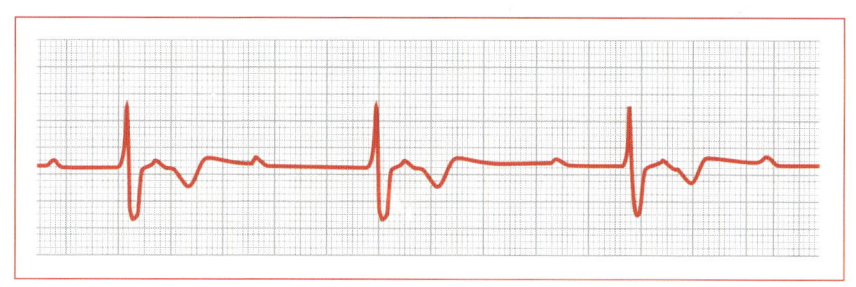

Figure 7. Electrocardiogram of third-degree atrioventricular block.

119

Chapter 8

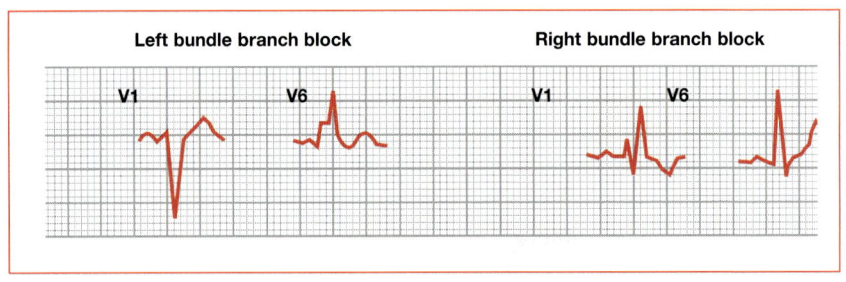

Figure 8. Electrocardiogram patterns of left bundle branch block and right bundle branch block.

Bundle branch block

A problem in the bundle of His presents in an identical fashion to a combined block of both bundles, ie, complete heart block. However, a more common occurrence is an isolated left or right bundle branch block. These are usually distinct from any problem with AV conduction (ie, they usually coexist with normal sinus rhythm [SR]). The patterns of the ECG are characteristic, but highly variable; the hallmark is a wide QRS complex.

- In left bundle branch block (LBBB), the pattern is best detected in V6 where there is an "M" pattern, while in V1 there is a "W" pattern (see **Figure 8**).
- In right bundle branch block (RBBB), the pattern is best detected in V1 where there is an RSR complex, while in V6 there is a QRS complex (see **Figure 8**).

In fact, both LBBB and RBBB are found in the "normal" population. New LBBB is cause for concern, and if it can clearly be related to an acute episode of chest pain then it probably indicates MI. Both RBBB and LBBB probably indicate increased risk for cardiovascular disease; however, neither on its own is an indication for pacing.

Fascicular block

One confusing aspect of electrocardiology is the terminology used to describe blocks of the fascicles (see **Figure 9**). The confusion arises from the fact that the right bundle is included in the list of three fascicles:

- left anterior fascicle
- left posterior fascicle
- right bundle branch

Arrhythmia

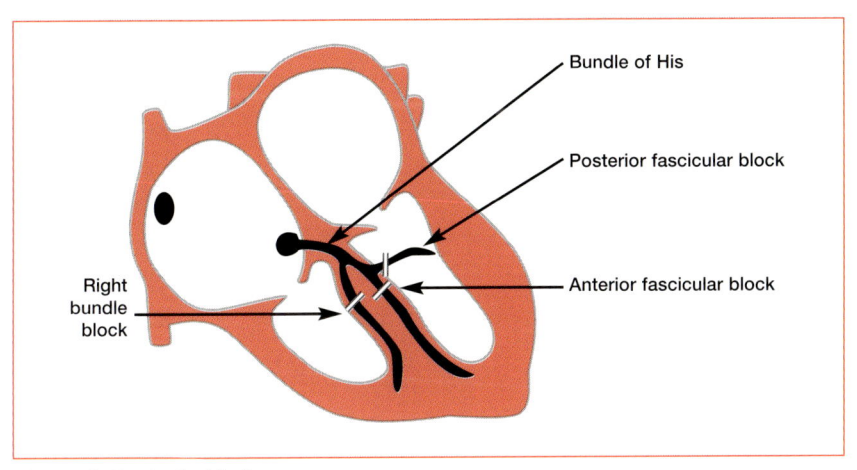

Figure 9. Fascicular block.

Left anterior and left posterior fascicular block
Fascicular block causes axis deviation on the ECG. Therefore, left anterior hemiblock causes left axis deviation (see **Figure 10**), while left posterior hemiblock causes right axis deviation (see **Figure 11**).

Bifascicular block
The term "bifascicular block" refers to a block of any two of the three fascicles. Clearly, this should include LBBB (left anterior + left posterior); however, the term is usually reserved for:

- RBBB + left anterior hemiblock, ie, RBBB + left axis deviation
- RBBB + left posterior hemiblock, ie, RBBB + right axis deviation
  (the axis is usually normal in RBBB)

Bifascicular block is not in itself an indication for pacing. However, when combined with intermittent second- or third-degree block, a DDD pacemaker should be fitted.

Trifascicular block
Trifascicular block refers to a block of all three fascicles (but with intact AV conduction). It usually refers to LBBB + a long PR interval. Although trifascicular block is not strictly speaking an indication for permanent pacing, some centers carry this out on the basis that it must reflect extensive conducting tissue damage.

Chapter 8

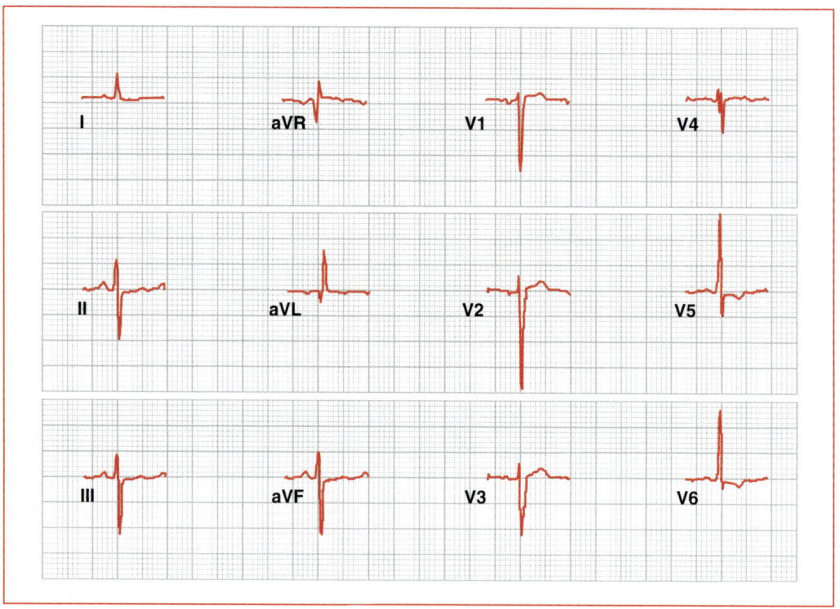

Figure 10. Left axis deviation.

Nonspecific intraventricular conduction defect
Another term that is sometimes used is "nonspecific intraventricular conduction defect". This usually refers to an abnormal ECG that does not clearly fit any of the patterns described above. The QRS complex will generally not be wide, but the waveform will be atypical. It is of unknown significance, but is likely to be benign.

Tachyarrhythmia

The general principle of patient management outlined at the beginning of this chapter holds true for patients suffering from tachyarrhythmia: is the patient compromised? And, as above, the use of an ECG will be critical when making the diagnosis. However, you will often be called to see a patient in the community where no ECG is available. In this situation, try to make a diagnosis based on the defibrillator monitor. Most patients with tachyarrhythmia will require referral, but making your own diagnosis can only help the situation. The key questions are:

- do the results show broad (>0.12 seconds) or narrow complexes?
- are they regular or irregular?

More sophisticated interpretation of the ECG is helpful, but the answers to these key questions will be sufficient to guide the immediate management (see **Table 5**).

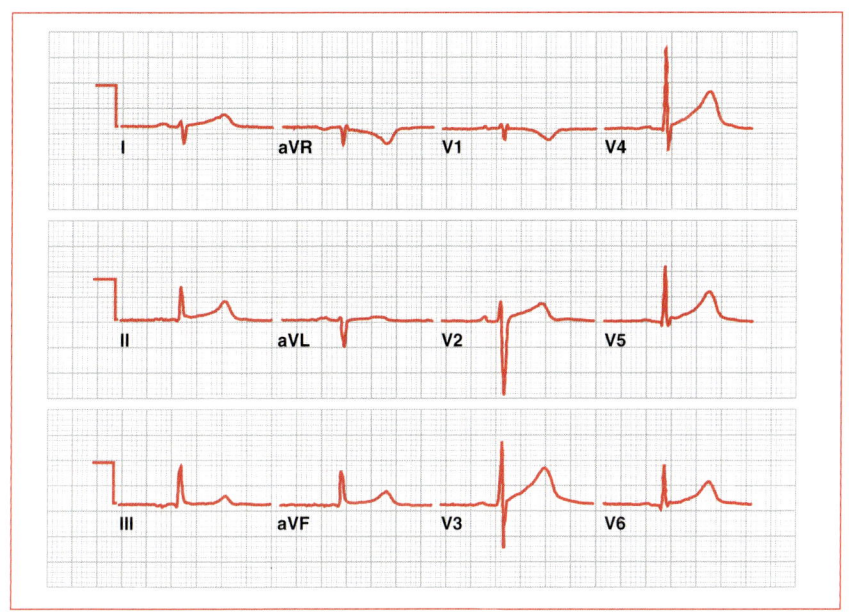

Figure 11. Right axis deviation.

Sinus tachycardia

Sinus tachycardia is usually a response to physiological stress such as exercise or anxiety, and it may be the result of an abnormally heightened sympathetic tone. Abnormal pathological causes include fever, hypotension, anemia, thyrotoxicosis, hypovolemia, pulmonary emboli, myocardial ischemia, and shock. Nicotine, caffeine, alcohol, and some medications (sympathetic agonists or parasympatholytic agents) are frequently the underlying cause of sinus tachycardia. The QRS complexes are preceded by P waves of normal morphology, duration, and axis. Sinus tachycardia alone does not require any treatment, but the underlying cause should be determined.

Atrial tachycardia

Atrial tachycardia can occur in the presence of cardiac or pulmonary disease at a rate varying from 140 to 240 bpm. P-wave morphology is generally different from that during SR, but the P–QRS relationship remains 1:1 (see **Figure 12**). Some atrial tachycardias are catecholamine sensitive; in this case, a β-blocker is appropriate therapy. Curative radiofrequency ablation of atrial tachycardia is effective in 70% of cases. For refractory cases, creation of complete heart block by radiofrequency catheter ablation with implantation of a permanent dual-chamber pacemaker provides control of the rate and avoids drug toxicity.

Chapter 8

Shape of complex	Diagnosis
Irregular narrow complex	Atrial fibrillation
	Atrial flutter (sawtooth pattern)
	Multifocal atrial tachycardia (distinct P waves, but with different morphologies)
Regular narrow complex	Sinus tachycardia
	Atrial flutter with constant AV block
	AVNRT
	Accessory pathway re-entrant tachycardia
Irregular broad complex	Atrial fibrillation + LBBB/RBBB
	Atrial fibrillation + other aberrant conduction
Regular broad complex	Sinus tachycardia + LBBB/RBBB
	Atrial flutter with constant AV block + LBBB/RBBB
	Ventricular tachycardia

Table 5. Possible diagnoses of tachyarrhythmias based on the electrocardiogram. AV: atrioventricular; AVNRT: atrioventricular nodal re-entrant tachycardia; LBBB: left bundle branch block; RBBB: right bundle branch block.

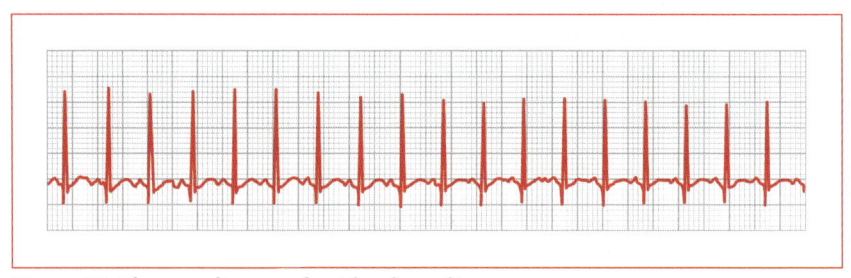

Figure 12. Electrocardiogram of atrial tachycardia.

Atrioventricular nodal re-entrant tachycardia

AV nodal re-entrant tachycardia (AVNRT) accounts for more than 70% of cases of paroxysmal SVT (see **Figures 13** and **14**). This is also termed "classic" SVT with fast (140–250 bpm) narrow complexes and no P waves. Initial management involves interventions to increase vagal tone. These should only be carried out on a monitored patient, and include:

- carotid sinus massage – apply firm pressure to one carotid artery at the level of the upper thyroid cartilage and move a small distance back and forth for up to 5 seconds (check for bruits first)
- Valsalva maneuver – the patient should take a deep breath, then attempt to exhale forcefully against a closed glottis for up to 15 seconds

Arrhythmia

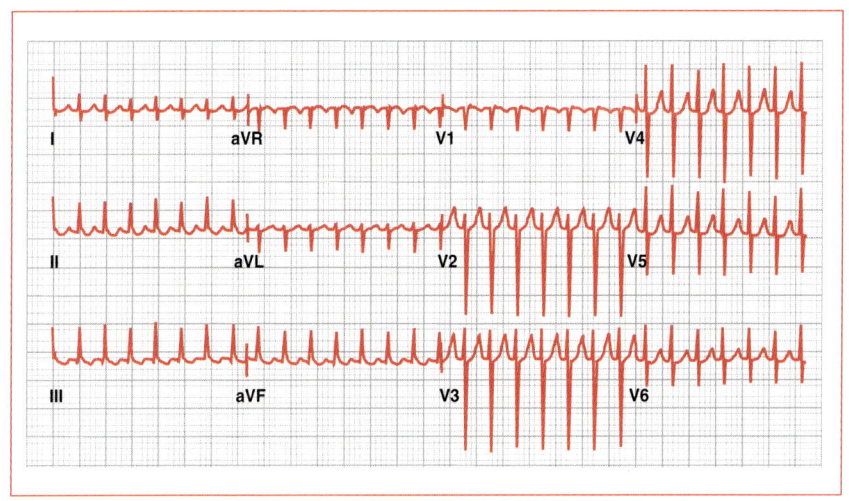

Figure 13. Electrocardiogram of atrioventricular nodal re-entrant tachycardia.

- diving reflex – this vestigial reflex, which allows marine animals to lower their metabolism when diving underwater, exists in humans and can increase vagal tone. Suddenly immerse the patient's face in very cold water

In a number of patients, the tachycardia (ie, AVNRT) terminates spontaneously with these maneuvers. However, if it does not, you should consider an adenosine challenge. This procedure involves rapid IV injections of increasing doses of adenosine (3–16 mg). Adenosine has a very short half-life (10 seconds) and produces temporary AV block, which can interrupt re-entry. This procedure is also very useful diagnostically, as the transient AV block can unmask an underlying atrial rhythm.

The use of a short-acting β-blocker (eg, esmolol) or a calcium-channel blocker (eg, verapamil) has also been found to be safe and effective in terminating AVNRT. Verapamil is particularly useful in patients with asthma, in whom adenosine is contraindicated.

Symptomatic patients with frequent episodes of AVNRT can be considered for radiofrequency catheter ablation of the "slow" pathway; this can be successfully ablated in more than 95% of cases.

Ventricular pre-excitation

Pre-excitation is defined as an early depolarization of the ventricular myocardium that occurs prior to any conduction through the AV node. The most common condition in which this is seen is WPW syndrome, where there is an accessory AV

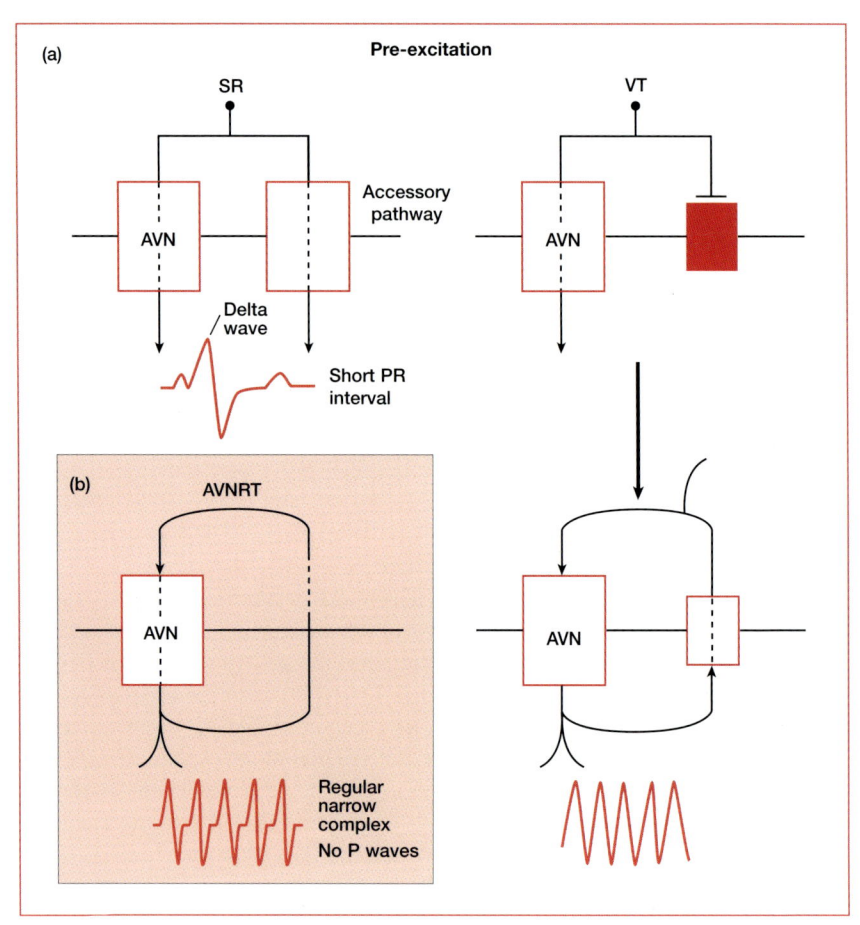

Figure 14. Mechanisms of re-entrant tachycardia. AVN: atrioventricular node; AVNRT: atrioventricular nodal re-entrant tachycardia; SR: sinus rhythm; VT: ventricular tachycardia.

pathway called the bundle of Kent. The anomalous conducting system can be located anywhere around the mitral or tricuspid rings. Most WPW patients have no evidence of structural heart disease. In the majority of cases, there is only a single accessory connection and the electrophysiological properties of the anomalous pathway differ from those of the AV node. Conduction through the accessory connection is faster and is independent of the heart rate. Consequently, the ventricular myocardium is activated from two directions: through the normal system and through the accessory pathway. The resulting QRS complex is a product of fusion of the two distinct activation wavefronts. Since conduction over the accessory pathway is faster, the initial part of the QRS complex represents ventricular activation through this route (delta wave – see **Figure 15**).

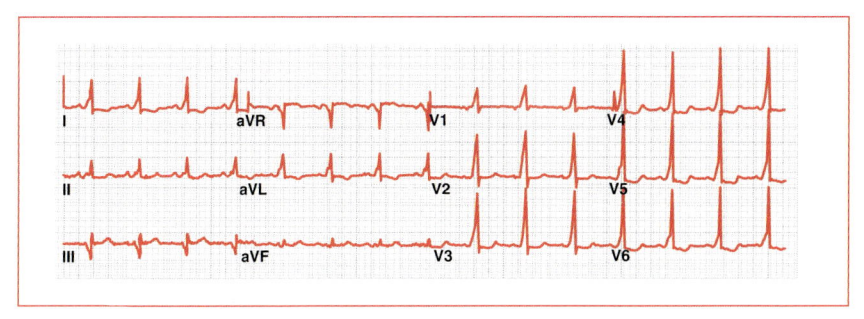

Figure 15. Electrocardiogram of Wolff–Parkinson–White syndrome.

The medical treatment of acute arrhythmias in WPW syndrome depends on the type of tachycardia. ECG results can help to determine this. A narrow complex indicates that accessory pathway re-entry is occurring. Treatment should include vagal maneuvers and adenosine as above. A broad complex is likely to be seen when AF is present, and can be particularly dangerous in WPW syndrome. It is characterized by rapid, irregular, wide complexes and should be treated by immediate direct current (DC) cardioversion. Adenosine, verapamil, and digoxin are not appropriate treatments as they increase the possibility of VT.

Following acute therapy, radiofrequency catheter ablation can be used as a curative treatment for symptomatic patients with an accessory pathway. Pathways can be successfully ablated in more than 90% of all cases and the recurrence rate after successful ablation is approximately 8%–10%. Severe complications are rare, occurring in 2% of all cases.

IN THE BEGINNING...
Wolff–Parkinson–White syndrome was first described by Frank Norman Wilson in 1915. Another case in a 19-year-old student was reported by Wedd in 1921, and Louis Wolff, John Parkinson, and Paul Dudley White alluded to these two descriptions when they described the disorder in 1930. The original article by these three authors contained an account of a form of bundle branch block in 11 healthy young adults who were subject to episodes of paroxysmal tachycardia. The relative contributions of the authors are uncertain. Wolff (1898–1972) and White (1886–1973) were both US cardiologists, while Parkinson (1885–1976) was an English physician: one patient had been seen at the London Hospital, while most of the others were examined in Boston. White was a giant of cardiology – he studied the ECG with Thomas Lewis and was a strong advocate of heart disease prevention through exercise, especially bicycle exercise. A bike path in Boston is named after him.

Chapter 8

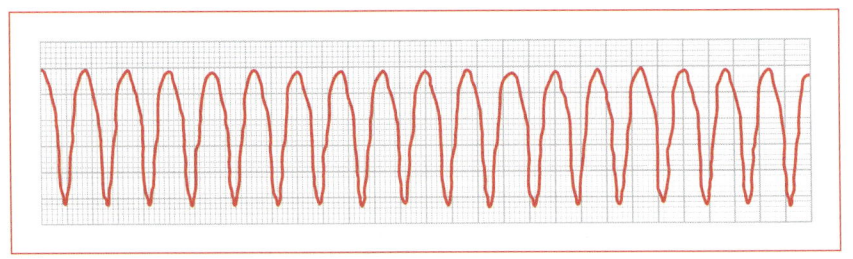

Figure 16. Electrocardiogram of ventricular tachycardia.

Ventricular tachycardia

In the acute situation, broad complex tachycardias present a diagnostic challenge because SVT with aberrant conduction can be difficult to distinguish from VT. As mentioned previously, the key question remains – is the patient compromised? Certain features on the ECG can help to distinguish VT from SVT (see **Figure 16**):

- a very broad QRS complex (>0.14 seconds)
- AV dissociation (but P waves are often difficult to distinguish in broad complex tachycardias)
- concordance (all QRS complexes in V1–V6 are either positive or negative)
- fusion beats
- capture beats

However, the key test is an adenosine challenge, which will interrupt an SVT but have no effect on VT. If VT is clear from the ECG or adenosine challenge has no effect and the patient is compromised, immediate DC cardioversion is needed. If there is time, a short-acting induction agent should be administered (or IV midazolam can be used). If the patient is losing consciousness, even this can be bypassed. Finally, if the patient loses their pulse, the cardiac arrest protocol should be immediately instituted (see Chapter 1, Cardiac arrest).

If the patient is only mildly compromised or suffering recurrent episodes, other therapeutic options are:

- IV amiodarone
- IV magnesium
- IV lidocaine (lignocaine) (no left ventricular [LV] dysfunction)
- overdrive pacing (this needs a temporary wire. The stimulator rate is turned up above the VT rate [usually ×3] to "capture" ventricular depolarization, and then gradually turned down)

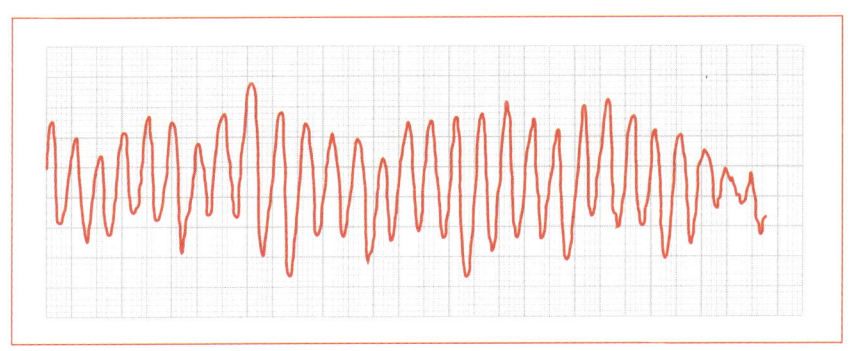

Figure 17. Electrocardiogram showing torsades de pointes.

The chronic investigation and management of VT will be carried out by a specialist (and probably a cardiologist with a special interest in electrophysiology). Investigation will center on finding a cause of VT. In the acute situation, there is often an obvious precipitating event (eg, MI). However, the most common cause of recurrent VT is ischemic heart disease. Another key aspect of the investigation will be distinguishing between polymorphic and monomorphic VT. The former, in which complexes vary within or between episodes in their pattern, has a stronger association with sudden death. In difficult cases of VT, invasive electrophysiological testing (often with concurrent coronary angiography) is warranted.

Control of chronic VT is pharmacological – typical drugs that are used include sotalol, flecainide, amiodarone, propafenone, and disopyramide – although radiofrequency ablation of the right ventricular (RV) outflow tract VT can be successful, and in some cases an automatic implantable cardioverter defibrillator (AICD) can save lives.

Ventricular ectopics

Ventricular ectopics, sometimes known as ventricular premature beats, are common in the general population. The shape of the complex is highly variable and depends on the ventricular source. Their significance is debated. They can be a marker of coronary disease and increased risk, but, without a precipitating cause, treatment generally does not lower risk. Electrolyte abnormalities should be excluded. If ventricular ectopics appear frequently during exercise (eg, an exercise tolerance test), the patient should be investigated further for coronary artery disease.

Torsades de pointes

This is a form of polymorphic VT that occurs when the SR shown on an ECG has a prolonged QT interval. The ECG exhibits a continuously changing axis (hence, "turning of points"; see **Figure 17**), which can look like ventricular fibrillation (VF). The prolonged QT interval can be caused by:

Chapter 8

Definition	Duration of atrial fibrillation
Paroxysmal	Up to 7 days
Persistent	Longer than 7 days
Permanent	Cardioversion failed or not attempted

Table 6. Classification of atrial fibrillation.

- antiarrhythmic agents
- hypokalemia
- hypomagnesemia
- bradycardia

However, in very rare cases it may be congenital (Jervell and Lange–Nielsen syndrome or Romano–Ward syndrome).

Atrial fibrillation

AF is the single most common cardiac arrhythmia. It is a condition where there is disorganized electrical and mechanical activity of the atria with a mechanism of multiple re-entrant wavelets. It may be chronic or occur in a paroxysmal fashion (see **Table 6**). On the ECG, it is recognized as an irregular rhythm with absent P waves (see **Figure 18**). Low-amplitude wavelets are frequently seen, but in many cases the baseline is flat. Usually, the ventricular response is controlled by the physiological conduction delay of the AV node and the ventricular response is slower in patients with diseases of the conducting system, in the elderly, or in individuals receiving medications that impair AV nodal conduction (eg, β-blockers, digitalis, or calcium-channel blockers). With intense sympathetic stimulation, it may be as rapid as 160–180 bpm.

The clinical manifestations of AF range from a complete absence of symptoms (usually in the young and fit) to hemodynamic collapse (in the elderly or those with systolic dysfunction). In addition to symptoms of palpitations, patients with AF have an increased risk of stroke and may also develop decreased exercise tolerance and LV dysfunction. The incidence of AF increases with age and its development is concentrated in patients with hypertensive heart disease, congestive heart failure, and rheumatic heart disease; the association with coronary artery disease is not as strong as with these other conditions. Among the noncardiac causes of AF, the association is strongest with hyperthyroidism, electrolyte abnormalities, and alcohol excess.

The patient with newly discovered AF

You will often be faced with a patient presenting with or without symptoms of AF, and an ECG showing the classic irregular rhythm with a flat or irregular baseline

Arrhythmia

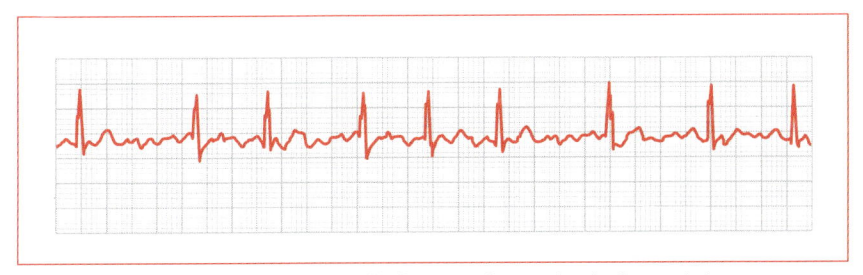

Figure 18. Electrocardiogram of atrial fibrillation with irregular rhythm and absent P waves.

(see **Figure 18**). The approach to management is guided, as before, by the clinical picture – is the patient compromised? If the answer is yes, you should refer immediately.

If not, you then have to decide whether the AF is persistent or paroxysmal (see **Figure 19**). A large proportion of patients experience spontaneous cardioversion within 24–48 hours of AF onset, but it is rarely clear whether this is their first episode. The best approach is to teach the patient to take his or her own pulse and monitor its regularity. This way, you can gain some idea of how long the patient spends in AF and in SR over the next few days.

If they spontaneously cardiovert, chronic treatment of paroxysmal AF takes three forms:

- anticoagulation
- rate control (if necessary)
- antiarrhythmics (the choice of which is guided by symptoms)

Most recent studies show that even patients with paroxysmal AF or successful cardioversion should remain on anticoagulation (warfarin, international normalized ratio [INR] 2–3) since these individuals have a greater risk of cerebrovascular events than of bleeding complications.

The use of rate control and antiarrhythmics is also individualized – some patients will require neither. However, a good choice is a beta-blocker (eg, carvedilol, metoprolol), which can impact both of these factors. Another choice for patients with heart failure or hypertension associated with AF is flecainide (in the absence of coronary artery disease) or amiodarone (if coronary artery disease is present).

If, several days following chronic treatment, patients remain in AF, there are two avenues of management: accept progression to permanent AF (and attend to rate control and anticoagulation) or attempt cardioversion.

Chapter 8

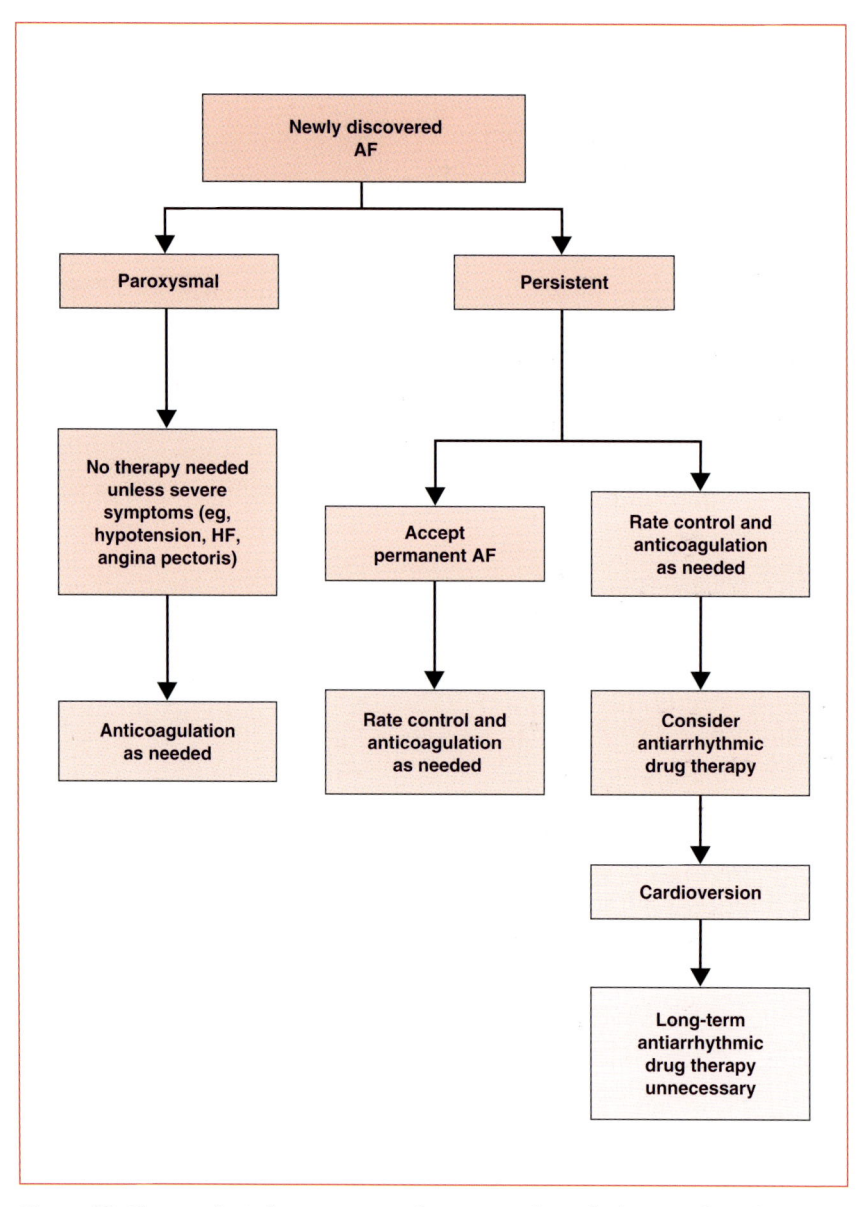

Figure 19. Pharmacological management of patients with newly discovered atrial fibrillation (AF). HF: heart failure. Reproduced with permission from the European Society of Cardiology (Fuster V, Ryden LE, Asinger RW. ACC/AHA/ESC Guidelines for the Managment of Patients with Atrial Fibrillation. *Eur Heart J* 2001;22:1852–923).

Deciding between the two (the decision will often be in the hands of the cardiologist) is influenced by several factors:

- How long has AF been present?
- How likely is SR to be maintained?
- What is the risk of thromboembolism?
- How severe are the symptoms?

Patients with longstanding AF or AF caused by structural abnormalities are least likely to stay in SR. Most cardiologists would agree that every patient should have one attempt at restoration of SR. However, this is not always the best policy. For example, in an elderly patient with asymptomatic, rate-controlled AF, the toxicity of antiarrhythmics may outweigh the benefit of restoration of SR.

The following points regarding treatment are helpful when treating a patient with AF.

- Regardless of the treatment strategy, all patients should have an ECG, chest x-ray, echo, and testing of thyroid function.
- If the decision is made to accept permanent AF, then control the rate with a combination of digoxin, a β-blocker, or a rate-limiting calcium-channel antagonist, and anticoagulate with warfarin, aiming for an INR of 2–3. The INR should be determined weekly (at least) in the initial stages and monthly thereafter. Patients over the age of 75 years who are considered at high risk for bleeding complications can be targeted to a lower INR of 2. In patients with contraindications to full anticoagulation, a daily dose of 300 mg aspirin can be used as an alternative to warfarin.
- If elective cardioversion is to be attempted, patients should be anticoagulated for 4 weeks with warfarin (aim for an INR of 2–3.5) and potassium levels should be kept in the upper normal range (>4.2 mmol) as this increases the chance of success of the cardioversion. Cardioversion can be electrical or chemical. If DC cardioversion is used, the patient receives a general anesthetic with a short-acting induction agent (usually propofol) and then receives shocks (synchronized to the R waves) of increasing energy: 100 J, 200 J, 360 J, and 360 J using paddles on the anterior and posterior chest (the patient lies on their side).

Chemical cardioversion is also possible using flecainide. In the event of successful cardioversion, patients should continue warfarin for at least 4 weeks. This is because the thromboembolic risk relates to "stunned" atria that do not resume normal mechanical function during this time.

Chapter 8

> **FAMOUS SCOTS**
> The first insight into the mechanism of irregular pulse in atrial fibrillation was provided by James Mackenzie, a Scottish GP who used an ink polygraph to record and label jugular venous pulses. He noticed that the jugular "a" wave was lost when patients went from a normal to an irregular rhythm.

New directions in the management of atrial fibrillation

It has recently been established that triggers in pulmonary veins can initiate AF and that circumferential or segmental disconnection of these veins at the left atrial junction can provide effective therapy. In certain patients, success rates for catheter-based pulmonary vein isolation range from 70% to 90%, but more than one procedure is often necessary. Surgery for AF is now usually reserved for use as an adjunctive treatment in patients having mitral or coronary surgery. Nevertheless, the large experience of the Maze procedure provides an important source of information to guide those performing catheter ablation. The Maze procedure was designed to exclude any place in the atria where the macro re-entrant circuits that underlie AF can form. Until recently, this involved an extensive series of atrial incisions, but the more recent cryosurgical Maze is just as effective and technically less demanding.

Atrial flutter

Atrial flutter is a rapid, regular rhythm with atrial rates of 250–350 bpm. The ventricular response rate varies, but it is usually a 2:1 block (creating the classic 150 bpm regular ventricular rhythm). The ECG pattern is typical – classic flutter waves are positive in the inferior leads and negative in lead V1 (see **Figure 20**).

Overall, atrial flutter is managed very much like AF:

- if the patient is hemodynamically compromised, one treatment option is DC cardioversion with low energy (50–100 J)
- a relatively easy way to convert atrial flutter to SR in the hospital setting is to use overdrive pacing in the high right atrium (RA)
- radiofrequency catheter ablation is now considered a curative approach in patients with recurrent atrial flutter. It can be eliminated by creating a linear lesion in the isthmus between the tricuspid annulus and the inferior vena cava. Acute success rates of 85%–90% and recurrence rates of 10%–15% have been reported
- patients with atrial flutter require anticoagulation therapy and, although there is more effective atrial contraction in atrial flutter (which may explain the decreased incidence of thromboembolism), guidelines are similar to those for AF

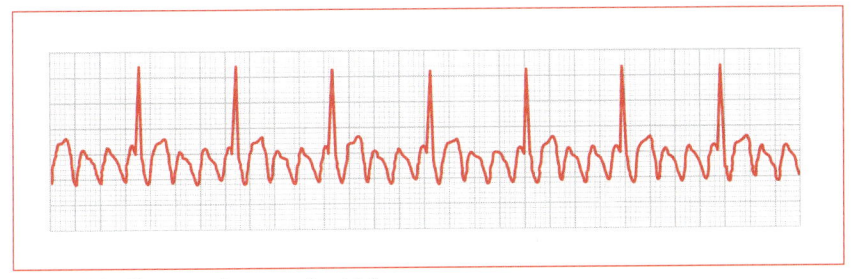

Figure 20. Electrocardiogram of atrial flutter.

Pacemakers

Implantation of a permanent electronic replacement for the heart's natural pacemaker began in the 1950s and is now a well-established treatment that increases patient longevity and improves their quality of life. Since its invention, advances in programmability, telemetry, and the ability to sense and pace two chambers have improved the level of care that can be provided. Miniaturization has made the process of implantation more straightforward and long-term complications less common. Advances in pacemaker technology mean that several new indications are likely to be added to the standard ones (see **Table 7**).

Pacemaker codes

Pacemaker codes are, to many, one of the most confusing aspects of electrocardiology (see **Table 8**). In fact, the labels, which are standardized, tell you all you need to know about the underlying programming and, in combination with the basic electrical wiring diagram of the heart (see **Figure 1**), can allow you to diagnose most problems.

The first letter refers to the chamber or chambers paced (atrium, ventricle, both [dual]). The second letter refers to the chamber sensed (atrium, ventricle, both [dual]) and the third letter details the response to sensing (triggered, inhibited, both [dual]). Thus, the most common pacemaker codes are the following.

(1) DDD – this box senses both chambers and if it detects a missing or late atrial or ventricular contraction it will pace one or both. The most common scenarios are:

- sinus bradycardia – atrial pacing will "kick in" and, assuming AV conduction is normal, no ventricular pacing will occur
- AV block (Mobitz type II; third-degree) – the ventricle is paced either following a normal atrial contraction or a paced atrial contraction. The benefit of this – that ventricular contraction will "track" the increased

Chapter 8

Indication	Pacemaker type	Clear consensus for indication
Sick sinus syndrome bradycardia	AAI, DDD	Yes
Carotid sinus syndrome syncope	DDI	Yes
Complete heart block (third-degree AV block)	DDD	Yes
Mobitz II block (second-degree AV block)	DDD	Yes
AF + AV block (pauses >3 seconds, ventricular rate <40 bpm)	VVI(R)	Yes
Trifascicular block	DDD	No
Malignant vasovagal syndrome	DDI	No

Table 7. Standard indications for pacemakers. AF: atrial fibrillation; AV: atrioventricular.

atrial rate of exercise tachycardia – is also its biggest drawback; it will also increase the ventricular pacing rate in the presence of abnormally increased atrial contraction, eg, atrial tachycardia

(2) VVI – this type of box is considerably cheaper than those boxes capable of DDD programming. It senses and paces only the ventricle and, consequently, only requires one lead. VVI boxes are indicated for use in AF with bradycardia and AV block, and in sinus bradycardia with no AV block. They can cause pacemaker syndrome and retrograde atrial tachycardia. They can also trigger AF.

(3) AAI – this device senses and paces only the atrium. It does not pace if a normal P wave is sensed. Thus, it is indicated for use in sick sinus syndrome to prevent bradycardia.

(4) Rate-adaptive pacemakers, eg, VVI(R). Some patients do not elevate their heart rate normally in response to exercise. This is known as chronotropic incompetence, and is defined as a failure to elevate the heart rate to 70% of predicted heart rate or to >100 bpm. It is most common in sick sinus syndrome (40% of cases), but it can also occur in AF. The solution to this condition is to use a rate-adaptive pacemaker. This type of pacemaker uses one of three methods to detect the need for an increased heart rate and responds accordingly. Examples of detection methods are: mechanical accelerometers that detect movement; changes in transthoracic impedance that can be used to detect changes in ventilation or RV filling; and QT sensors that respond to the shortening of the paced QT interval by catecholamines.

Paced	Sensed	Response	Rate
A	A	T	R
V	V	I	
D	D	D	

Table 8. Pacemaker codes. A: atrium; D: dual (ie, both chambers or both responses); I: inhibited; R: rate responsive; T: triggered; V: ventricle.

Implantation

Pacemaker implantation is carried out under sedation. Leads are inserted via the subclavian or cephalic vein into the RA and/or RV. Atrial leads are J-shaped and are positioned in the right atrial appendage (anteriorly and superiorly in the RA). Ventricular leads are positioned in the RV apex. Most ventricular leads are placed in position and left against the myocardial wall. In certain circumstances, eg, when these leads become easily displaced or do not provide adequate threshold values, an active fixation lead can be used. This lead has a screw "thread" on its end – usually covered by a dissolvable tip, so that it is not exposed until it is in position – that allows the lead to be fixed into the myocardium.

After the leads are positioned, a series of tests are carried out to determine if the lead position is satisfactory from an electrical point of view. These would typically assess:

- threshold
  - the voltage required to cause a contraction. This increases if the lead is not well-positioned and can be a sensitive method of detecting poor placement
- lead impedance
  - this is a test of the integrity of the lead. It is essentially a measure of electrical resistance and is measured in Ohms
- abnormal stimulation of the phrenic nerve
  - a high-voltage protocol tests for a diaphragmatic twitch

THE PACEMAKER'S MAKER

Canadian John Hopps invented the first cardiac pacemaker. Hopps was trained as an electrical engineer at the University of Manitoba and joined the National Research Council in 1941, where he conducted research on hypothermia. While experimenting with radiofrequency heating to restore body temperature, Hopps made an unexpected discovery: if a heart stopped beating due to cooling, it could be started again by artificial stimulation using mechanical or electrical means. In 1950, this led to Hopps' invention of the world's first cardiac pacemaker. His device was far too large to be implanted inside the human body – it was an external pacemaker.

Once all the required tests are completed, the pacemaker pocket (in the fascia overlying the pectoral muscle) is created by blunt dissection and the wound sutured.

Complications

Acute complications will generally occur in hospital. These may include pneumothorax, RV perforation and cardiac tamponade, and hematoma.

Chronic complications are more likely to present to the generalist. Lead infection is fortunately rare, but can present a very difficult management problem. Skin commensals are the most common culprits in right-sided endocarditis. If you suspect this, you should immediately refer the patient for an echo and blood cultures. Treatment is initially with antibiotics, but the lead system should be quickly replaced if this is unsuccessful.

Lead displacement can occur as a result of concurrent right-sided pathology, eg, RV dilatation or valve abnormalities, and can be detected by changes in threshold. Changes in impedance can point to deterioration of old wires or loss of insulation properties. Subclavian vein or superior vena cava occlusion is more common with multiple lead systems. Classic signs include unilateral superficial vein engorgement around the upper thorax, neck, and face.

Erosion occasionally occurs if the pacemaker box becomes gradually more superficial. Unless it causes chronic pain, or erodes completely, it does not demand referral. Some patients move their own box back and forward under the skin (Twiddler's syndrome). This can cause hemorrhage or lead breaks.

Infection of the implantation site can be problematic and should be taken seriously. In the early stage, superficial redness of the skin or swelling around the box will be noticed. For this, standard treatment is indicated, eg, a skin swab, cloxacillin (flucloxacillin) (oral dosage, 500 mg four times daily). If the infection does not respond, or if you suspect deep infection for another reason, eg, marked constitutional symptoms, refer immediately. Infections resistant to antibiotic therapy demand box and lead extraction – a procedure not without difficulty or complications.

Pacemaker syndrome occurs in some patients with a VVI pacemaker who are in SR. It is thought to relate to the fact that although sometimes the atria contract "in time" and cardiac output is normal, at other times they contract against closed AV valves, which causes elevated venous pressure and a fall in cardiac output. The patient will experience dizziness, and the solution is to upgrade the patient to a DDD pacemaker.

Finally, atrial-sensing pacemakers, eg, DDD, respond to atrial arrhythmia with tachycardic pacing. If this happens, it is possible to alter the program (to DDI or set an upper rate limit) or use antiarrhythmic drugs. This problem can be avoided by using a mode-switching pacemaker that detects atrial arrhythmia and switches to VVI.

Pacemaker ECGs
ECGs are harder to interpret in a patient with a pacemaker as there are more variables; although the pacing spikes are usually straightforward to recognize. It is important to remember that the paced QRS complex will be in an LBBB pattern because the wave of depolarization begins where the lead is placed in the RV.

Doctor, I have a pacemaker, what should I avoid?
This is a common question that patients ask. In general, patients should live life as normal. They should avoid magnetic resonance imaging studies, and care should be taken with the following:

- electrocautery during surgery – this can cause sensing problems
- therapeutic radiation
- cardioversion/defibrillation – this should be carried out using the lowest effective energy with the paddles in the anterior–posterior positions on the body of the patient
- mobile phones – these should not be placed in a shirt pocket next to the pacemaker
- car batteries – batteries can produce large magnetic fields. Again, this is only a problem if the person is leaning over and the pacemaker comes close to the battery
- high-voltage cables

Most manufacturers supply each pacemaker recipient with a wallet-sized emergency card for identification as the bearer of an implanted device. This card should include important information about current pacing parameters, names and numbers of the pulse generator (including leads), indication for pacing, and underlying structural heart disease.

Patient follow-up
Application of a magnet to many pacemaker generators reveals the current battery status by pacing with a fixed pacing rate or "magnet rate". The pacemaker rate decreases in most models with declining battery charge. When a decrease indicates exhaustion of one battery capacity, the pulse generator should be replaced.

Implantable cardioverter defibrillators

The natural evolution of pacemaker technology led, in the late 1960s, to the development of the AICD. Early versions were implanted abdominally under general anesthesia. These boxes, now barely bigger than a VVI pacemaker, are implanted under heavy sedation/light general anesthesia, and have revolutionized the treatment of ventricular arrhythmias. Indications for use of the device are expanding as the evidence base grows, but at present these include VF or VT cardiac arrest without a reversible cause; spontaneous sustained VT; syncope of undetermined origin with hemodynamically significant sustained VT; and nonsustained VT with prior MI or LV dysfunction. A recent study suggested that all post-MI patients with an EF <30% should receive an ACD.

An AICD is expensive – approximately the same cost as bypass grafting – but the device is multifunctional. It is capable of bradycardia and tachyarrhythmia detection, overdrive pacing or defibrillation, and event memory (ie, it can "play back" the intracardiac trace from a few minutes before the event, which is extremely useful diagnostically).

The AICD contains a device program for termination of VT and this highlights its versatility. It can initiate:

- burst pacing – a short burst of paced beats delivered at approximately 90% of the rate of the VT
- ramp pacing – a short burst of paced beats at a rate increasing up to 90% of the rate of the VT (to try to achieve capture)
- low-energy shock
- high-energy shock

The programming of AICDs is sophisticated and is carried out by telemetry (a magnet detector is placed over the unit). The energy of shock delivered by the AICD is a magnitude less than that delivered across the chest wall by an external defibrillator (internal 5–35 J, external 100–360 J). If an AICD delivers a shock, it is important to refer the patient to the nearest center where the unit can be interrogated.

Electrophysiological studies

Electrophysiology is a rapidly advancing field in which the potential indications currently outweigh the availability of facilities. The indications for electrophysiology are detailed in **Table 9**.

The essence of the electrophysiological test is a measurement of the intracardiac ECG: (1) during normal SR; (2) during an induced arrhythmia; and (3) following premature extrastimuli.

Arrhythmia

Potential indications for electrophysiology
Sinus node dysfunction • to evaluate the AV node or where the link between symptoms and arrhythmia is not secure
AV block • suspected infranodal block (ie, pathology of the bundle of His or Purkinje fibers) • intraventricular conduction delay
Frequent AVNRT • especially if frequent episodes occur despite drug treatment
Wolff–Parkinson–White syndrome • to characterize the accessory pathway and ablate it
Unexplained syncope • after a negative tilt test, or in the presence of known heart disease
Cardiac arrest • in the absence of myocardial infarction

Table 9. Potential indications for electrophysiology. AV: atrioventricular; AVNRT: atrioventricular nodal re-entrant tachycardia.

Class	Typically	Mechanism	Action potential duration	Uses
1a	Quinidine, procainamide, disopyramide	Block sodium channels (short dissociation time)	↑	Supraventricular and ventricular tachycardias Rarely used
1b	Lidocaine (lignocaine)	Block sodium channels (medium dissociation time)	↓	Ventricular tachycardias Used post-MI
1c	Flecainide, propafenone	Block sodium channels (long dissociation time)	↔	Ventricular tachycardia
2	β-blockers, (eg, atenolol)	Abrogate sympathetic drive	↔	Commonly used for ventricular and supraventricular arrhythmias post-MI
3	Amiodarone, sotalol	Inhibit potassium current	↑	Commonly used for ventricular and supraventricular arrhythmias
4	Diltiazem, verapamil	Block L-type calcium channels	Block at AV node	Ventricular rate control Termination of SVT

Table 10. The Vaughan-Williams classification of antiarrhythmic drugs.
AV: atrioventricular; MI: myocardial infarction; SVT: supraventricular tachycardia; ↑: increase in duration; ↓: decrease in duration; ↔: no change in duration.

Chapter 8

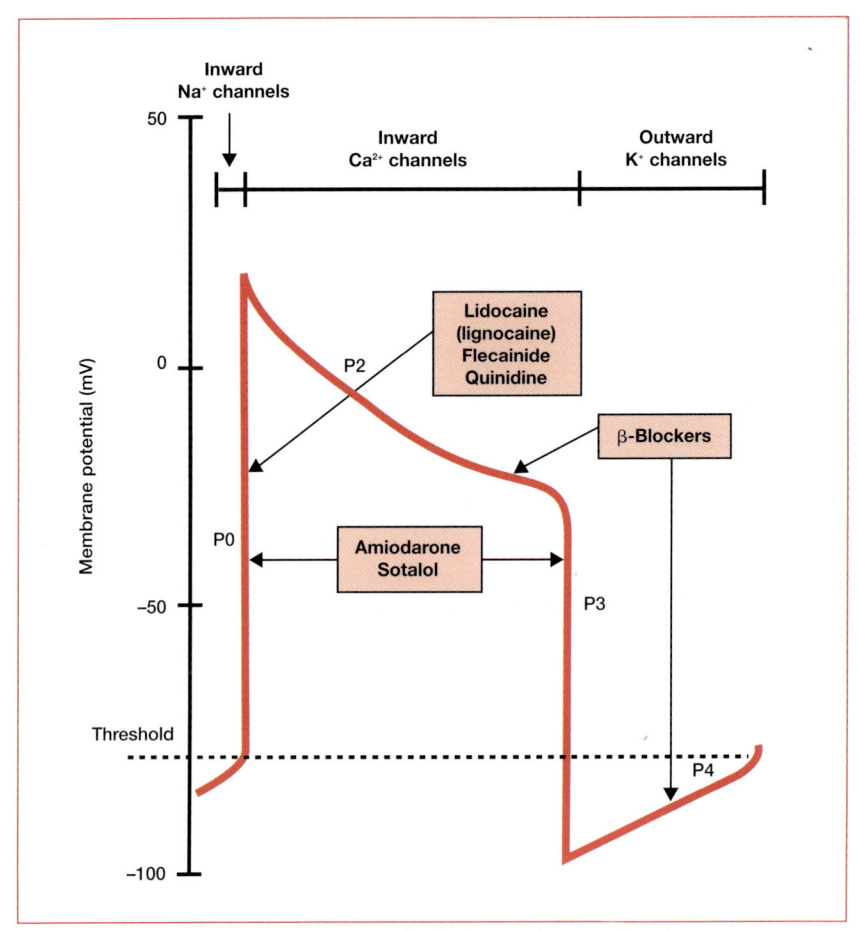

Figure 21. Drugs used in the treatment of arrhythmia. The typical cardiac action potential is also shown: a fast sodium current and slower calcium current depolarize cardiac cells. The plateau phase caused by calcium entry contributes to the long refractory period, which protects the heart from re-excitation.

Measurements are usually taken from several intracardiac sites, allowing identification of sinus node function and recovery, sinoatrial conduction, AV nodal conduction, and triggered ventricular arrhythmias. Treatment is with radiofrequency stimulation, which can ablate accessory pathways or interrupt re-entry circuits.

Drugs in arrhythmia

Table 10 describes the Vaughan-Williams classification of antiarrhythmic drugs, and **Figure 21** outlines the drugs used in the treatment of arrhythmia.

Further reading

Fuster V, Ryden LE, Asinger RW et al. ACC/AHA/ESC Guidelines for the Management of Patients With Atrial Fibrillation: Executive Summary. A Report of the American College of Cardiology/American Heart Association Task Force on Practice Guidelines and the European Society of Cardiology Committee for Practice Guidelines and Policy Conferences (Committee to Develop Guidelines for the Management of Patients With Atrial Fibrillation) Developed in collaboration with the North American Society of Pacing and Electrophysiology. *Eur Heart J* 2001;22:1852–923.

Guidelines for Clinical Intracardiac Electrophysiological and Catheter Ablation Procedures. A report of the American College of Cardiology/American Heart Association Task Force on practice guidelines. (Committee on Clinical Intracardiac Electrophysiologic and Catheter Ablation Procedures). Developed in collaboration with the North American Society of Pacing and Electrophysiology. *Circulation* 1995;92:673–91.

Silverman ME. From rebellious palpitations to the discovery of auricular fibrillation: contributions of Mackenzie, Lewis and Einthoven. *Am J Cardiol* 1994;73:384–9.

Wolff L, Parkinson J, White PD. Bundle-branch block with short P-R interval in healthy young people prone to paroxysmal tachyardia. *Am Heart J* 1930;5:685.

Chapter 9

Valve disease

Disease of the heart valves remains an important cause of morbidity and mortality across the world. While advances in echocardiography and the widespread availability of antibiotics have changed the prevalence, management, and especially the diagnosis of valve disease for specialists, very little has changed for generalists, who hear heart murmurs less frequently. Even though echo diagnosis is not readily available to generalists, they nevertheless feel pressured to identify murmurs and to report them, with their associated signs, in the referral letter. Similarly, for many examiners, the appeal of obscure murmurs for clinical short-case exams remains too great to resist, despite its mostly historical relevance. Yet, there are few greater pleasures in clinical medicine than having your stethoscopic diagnostic brilliance confirmed by an echo report. Furthermore, healthcare economics has prompted a renewed interest in the power of the stethoscope for diagnosing and even quantifying valve disease.

The asymptomatic murmur

Opinions differ as to the management of a murmur that has been picked up incidentally. By far the most common is the mid systolic 2/6 murmur (grade II – see **Table 1**). For children and young adults with an asymptomatic mid systolic murmur, a negative history and a negative physical exam are sufficient to exclude sinister pathology in most cases.

Grade	Murmur
I	Just audible in a quiet room
II	Quiet
III	Loud, no thrill
IV	Loud, with thrill
V	Very loud with thrill
VI	Audible without a stethoscope

Table 1. Grading of murmurs.

Chapter 9

In the elderly, it is important to differentiate between the common and benign aortic sclerosis and the less common and less benign aortic stenosis (AS). As such, close attention should be paid to the cardiac exam. In particular, AS is indicated by:

- murmur radiation
- the presence of a thrill
- a soft second heart sound

In addition, an electrocardiogram should be carried out to screen for left ventricular hypertrophy (LVH), ischemia, and atrial size or conduction abnormalities. If none of the above is present and the patient remains asymptomatic, the most likely diagnosis is aortic sclerosis and no echo is required.

Referral is warranted when a murmur in an asymptomatic patient is:

- systolic and grade III or above
- late systolic
- mid systolic and accompanied by clinical signs suggestive of AS
- diastolic
- continuous

Aortic stenosis

Causes
Congenital aortic stenosis
Congenital AS is usually due to a bicuspid valve. A bicuspid valve in itself does not give rise to significant hemodynamic abnormality, but it has a tendency to calcify and a predisposition to infective endocarditis (see **Table 2**).

Rheumatic aortic stenosis
Rheumatic AS results from cusp fusion and calcification many years following rheumatic fever.

Senile aortic stenosis
Senile, or degenerative, AS results from calcium deposition on the aortic surface of the valve. This is becoming an increasingly important disability problem in the elderly.

Physical signs

- The carotid pulse is slow rising with reduced amplitude.
- The venous pressure is usually normal until late in the disease.

Valve disease

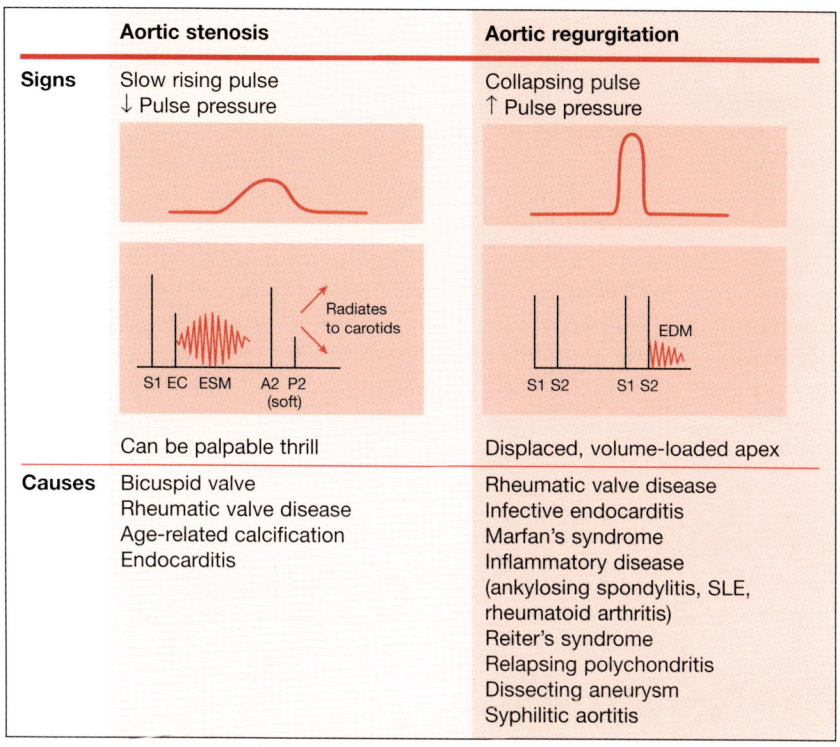

	Aortic stenosis	Aortic regurgitation
Signs	Slow rising pulse ↓ Pulse pressure S1 EC ESM A2 P2 (soft) Radiates to carotids Can be palpable thrill	Collapsing pulse ↑ Pulse pressure S1 S2 S1 S2 EDM Displaced, volume-loaded apex
Causes	Bicuspid valve Rheumatic valve disease Age-related calcification Endocarditis	Rheumatic valve disease Infective endocarditis Marfan's syndrome Inflammatory disease (ankylosing spondylitis, SLE, rheumatoid arthritis) Reiter's syndrome Relapsing polychondritis Dissecting aneurysm Syphilitic aortitis

Table 2. Clinical signs in aortic stenosis and aortic regurgitation. EC: ejection click; EDM: early diastolic murmur; ESM: ejection systolic murmur; SLE: systemic lupus erythematosus.

- The apex beat is sustained and can be doubled due to an additional atrial component.
- On auscultation, the second heart sound is single when the valve is calcified due to a lack of aortic component. The classic ejection systolic murmur, which can radiate to one or both carotids, is usually heard best over the aortic area. A soft, early diastolic murmur of aortic regurgitation (AR) often coexists.

Investigation and management

Echo is the diagnostic tool of choice for valve disease – in particular, Doppler measurement of valve gradients can quantify lesions. Significant hemodynamic changes do not occur until the aortic valve area has been reduced to a quarter of its normal size (the normal orifice is 3–4 cm^2). AS is classed as:

- mild if the area is >1.5 cm^2
- moderate if the area is 1–1.5 cm^2
- severe if the area is <1 cm^2

Chapter 9

> **THE INVENTION OF THE STETHOSCOPE**
> "In the summer of 1816, Laennec was called to a young lady who presented the general symptoms of disease of the heart; the application of the hand to the chest and percussion afforded very little assistance, and immediate auscultation was interdicted by the sex and embonpoint[a] of the patient. The recollection of the well-known fact, that the tap of a pin at one end of a beam could be heard distinctly at the opposite end, induced him at the moment, to avail himself of this acoustic phenomenon. He took a quire of paper, rolled it tightly together, applied one extremity over the region of the heart, and putting the ear to the other, was surprised to find that he could distinguish the pulsation of the heart in a more distinct manner than he could before do with the naked ear. Having hit upon the principle he extended its application to the investigation of the various sounds produced in the chest by the respiration, the voice, and the accidental presence of fluids in the lung, pleural sac, and pericardium."
> Mediate Auscultation, 1816. (Quoted in The Lancet 1998;352:997.)
> [a]Corpulence, physically bulky.

Severe stenosis causes a transvalvular pressure gradient of >50 mm Hg in the presence of normal transvalvular flow (ie, normal LV function). However, abnormally low pressure gradients are found in conditions of LV dysfunction, so the gradient alone is not a clear guide.

The natural history of AS is one of slow progression. Studies suggest that some patients exhibit a decrease in valve area of 0.1–0.3 cm^2/year, although no progression is discernible in many patients. However, regardless of the individual variability, symptoms of angina, syncope, or heart failure generally develop after a latent period. At this point, the outlook changes dramatically. After the onset of symptoms, the average survival is less than 3 years. Thus, development of symptoms is the critical point in the natural history of AS and thereafter the benefits of surgery outweigh the risk. Consequently, asymptomatic AS patients should be monitored closely. Although there is no clear consensus, most cardiologists follow-up mild AS annually (together with 5-yearly echos); moderate AS every 6 months (together with 2-yearly echos); and severe AS more frequently (together with annual echos). If a patient with AS presents with a change in symptoms, their next appointment at the cardiology clinic should be expedited.

If a patient with severe AS is undergoing open chest bypass grafting for coexisting coronary artery disease (CAD), the opportunity should be taken to carry out aortic valve replacement (AVR) – regardless of whether or not AS symptoms are evident. The merit of carrying out a concomitant AVR is less clear for those with mild or moderate AS.

Cardiac catheterization is only indicated in AS for two reasons: (1) to perform coronary angiography before AVR in patients with risk factors for CAD; (2) to assess the severity of AS in symptomatic patients when AVR is planned or when noninvasive tests are inconclusive (catheterization allows accurate quantification of the orifice because it can account for transvalvular flow).

Contrary to popular belief, exercise testing is not contraindicated for mild to moderate AS patients and can give useful information with respect to exercise capacity, heart rate recovery, and exercise-induced rise in blood pressure.

Balloon valvotomy
Percutaneous balloon aortic valvotomy (stretching a stenotic valve by balloon inflation) has an important role to play in the treatment of young adults with AS, but a very limited role in older patients. This is because the postoperative valve area is rarely >1 cm^2 and because complications are frequent (10%) and serious. This procedure can act as a "bridge" to reduce the requirement for surgery (with its inherent risk) in adult patients with refractory pulmonary edema or cardiogenic shock.

Aortic valve replacement in the elderly
Due to the limitations of medical therapy and balloon valvotomy, AVR should be considered for all elderly patients with symptomatic AS. However, the decision as to whether to carry out AVR is rarely straightforward and must take into account the risks as viewed by both the surgeon and the patient. Comorbidity in the form of LVH or CAD greatly increases the risk associated with surgery. In addition, specific valve problems, such as heavy calcification and narrow LV outflow tract or annulus, make the procedure more complex. The decision is highly individual.

Aortic regurgitation

AR is associated with classic clinical signs (see **Table 2**):

- waterhammer (collapsing) pulse – detected by comparing the character of the radial pulse at the level of the heart with its character on elevation of the arm (use several fingers). Elevation accentuates the steep rise-and-fall character of this pulse, which seems to slap faster and harder against the fingers
- Corrigan's sign – visible arterial pulsation in the neck
- de Musset's sign – nodding of the head in time with the heartbeat
- Duroziez's sign – caused by retrograde diastolic flow in the femoral artery. Place the stethoscope on the femoral pulse and occlude the artery distally. The turbulent flow will be picked up as a "to-and-fro" murmur

- Quincke's sign – capillary pulsation in the nail beds that is visible on applying gentle pressure to induce a degree of whitening
- Traube's sign – a "pistol-shot" sound heard over the femoral pulse
- Müller's sign – pulsation of the uvula

An early diastolic murmur is heard at the left lower sternal edge when the patient is sitting forward and holding his or her breath in expiration. There could also be a coexistent aortic systolic flow murmur, caused by the large stroke volume (rather than reflecting organic AS). There may be a mid diastolic murmur at the apex (Austin Flint murmur) caused by the regurgitant aortic jet vibrating the anterior mitral valve (MV) leaflet.

Acute aortic regurgitation

Acute AR is one hallmark of aortic dissection and is a medical emergency in its own right. A large regurgitant volume is suddenly imposed on an LV of normal size that has not had time to accommodate to the volume overload. The result is a reduction in stroke volume, compensatory tachycardia, pulmonary edema, and cardiogenic shock. Characteristic clinical findings are absent and an echo is essential to document the severity of the lesion. This is done by assessing the speed of equilibration of aortic and LV pressures in diastole. Useful echo measures are short regurgitant wave half time, short mitral deceleration time, and premature closure of the MV.

Mortality is high in acute severe AR and early surgical intervention is essential. Nitroprusside can be helpful in reducing preload and afterload, possibly in combination with dobutamine or dopamine. Intra-aortic balloon pumping is absolutely contraindicated (it increases aortic diastolic pressure and worsens the regurgitation), while β-blockers, often used in the management of dissection, should be used with caution in associated acute severe AR as they dampen the compensatory tachycardia.

Chronic aortic regurgitation

An early diastolic murmur is always justification for referral to a cardiologist for assessment and echo.

Causes

- Rheumatic involvement of the aortic valve, resulting in thickening of the cusps and fusion of the commissures – the valve neither opens nor closes completely.
- Dilatation of the aortic root resulting from aneurysm of the ascending aorta – this is commonly seen in Marfan's syndrome.

- Dilatation of the aortic annulus can also result from connective tissue disease, such as ankylosing spondylitis, rheumatoid arthritis, Reiter's syndrome, relapsing polychondritis, or systemic lupus erythematosus.
- Dissecting aneurysm involving the aortic root.
- Syphilitic aortitis causing aortic aneurysm and dilatation of the valve ring that may involve the coronary ostia.

Table 2 outlines the causes of aortic regurgitation.

Natural history and therapeutic options
Chronic AR represents a condition of combined volume and pressure overload on the LV. The ejection fraction (EF) – the percentage of the end diastolic volume ejected during systole – is maintained by compensatory LVH and the majority of patients remain in this compensated phase for decades. However, in time, the EF drops. Although initially this is fully reversible, soon, due to progressive dilatation and remodeling, full recovery with AVR is out of reach. A large number of studies have identified LV systolic dysfunction and end systolic dimension as the key determinants of survival in patients undergoing AVR for AR. Thus, in contrast to AS, the critical point when the benefit of AVR outweighs the risk is determined not by symptoms, but by echo-determined LV function. More specifically, AVR is indicated in:

- patients with New York Heart Association (NYHA) class III or IV symptoms (see Chapter 7, Heart failure) and preserved LV systolic function – defined as normal EF ($\geq$50% at rest)
- patients with NYHA class II symptoms and preserved LV systolic function at rest, but with progressive LV dilatation, declining rest EF, or declining effort tolerance (the trend is more important than the absolute level)
- patients with angina on walking or climbing stairs rapidly
- asymptomatic or symptomatic patients with mild to moderate LV dysfunction at rest (EF 25%–49%)
- patients undergoing open chest surgery for another reason (eg, bypass grafting)

Exercise testing can be useful in AR if the patient is sedentary or has equivocal symptoms. It assesses functional capacity and the hemodynamic effects of exercise. Radionuclide ventriculography should be used if the echo window is poor. Cardiac catheterization is only required in patients at risk of CAD prior to AVR or where other tests are equivocal.

Asymptomatic patients with no LV dysfunction should be encouraged to participate in all forms of normal daily activity, including exercise (although lifting weights should be avoided).

Vasodilator therapy can, in theory, retard the natural history of chronic AR by reducing the regurgitant volume. However, very few studies have actually examined the effect of this treatment on the long-term outcome. Indications for vasodilator therapy (generally using long-acting nifedipine) are:

- long-term therapy in patients with severe regurgitation who have symptoms and/or LV dysfunction, when surgery is not recommended
- long-term therapy in asymptomatic patients with severe regurgitation who have LV dilatation, but normal systolic function
- long-term therapy in asymptomatic patients with hypertension and any degree of regurgitation
- long-term therapy in patients with persistent LV systolic dysfunction after AVR (angiotensin-converting enzyme inhibitor)
- short-term therapy to improve the hemodynamic profile of patients with severe heart failure symptoms and severe LV dysfunction before proceeding with AVR

Asymptomatic patients with mild AR and normal LV systolic function should be seen by a cardiologist annually and undergo echo every 2–3 years. Asymptomatic patients with normal systolic function, but severe AR and significant LV dilatation (end diastolic diameter >6 cm), require more frequent evaluation. These patients should be seen by a cardiologist every 6 months and undergo echo every 6–12 months.

Mitral stenosis

The MV apparatus consists of three components: two leaflets, the fibrous annulus, and the chordae tendineae, which connect the leaflets to the papillary muscles (see **Figure 1**). The anterior leaflet is larger than the posterior leaflet (see **Figure 2**). The normal area of the MV orifice is 4–5 cm^2. Symptoms of mitral stenosis (MS) develop when the orifice is <2.5 cm^2 and a critical stenosis occurs when it is approximately 1 cm^2 (see **Figure 3**). The signs and causes of MS are outlined in **Table 3**.

Causes
Rheumatic heart disease is the most common cause of MS, although it pre-dates the symptoms by at least 10 years. Other acquired causes are rare – eg, annular calcification, endocarditis, or granulomatous infiltration in association with eosinophilia.

Valve disease

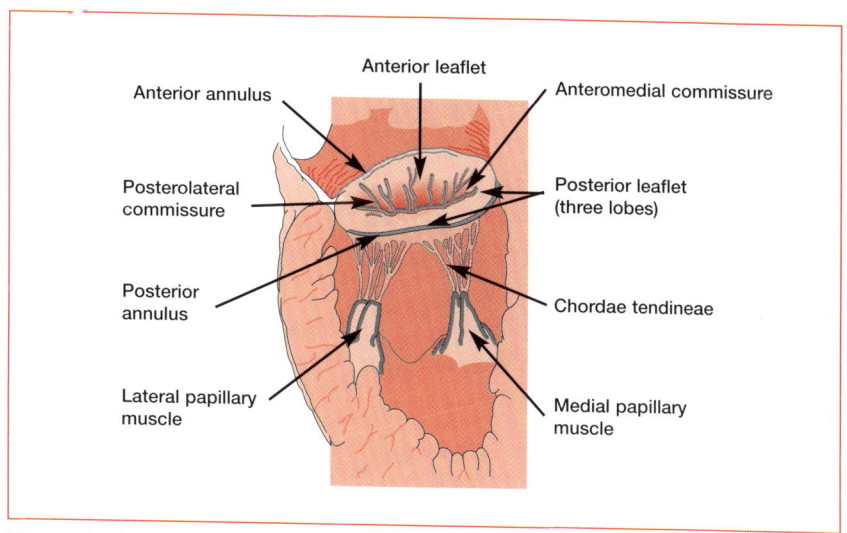

Figure 1. The structure of the mitral valve apparatus.

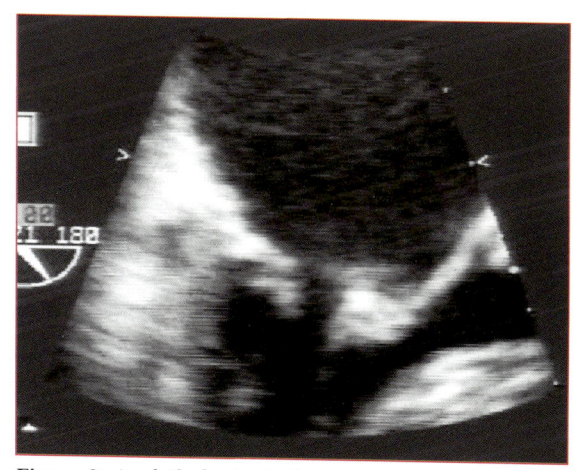

Figure 2. A calcified mitral valve posterior leaflet in diastole.

Signs

Symptoms of MS generally occur during exertion, infection, stress, or with the onset of atrial fibrillation (AF) with a rapid ventricular response. This is because a left atrial (LA) pressure that is normal at rest rises with an increase in transmitral flow or a decrease in the diastolic filling time.

The most common manifestation is breathlessness, but a reduction in exercise tolerance or symptoms of right-sided congestion can also occur. The typical

153

Chapter 9

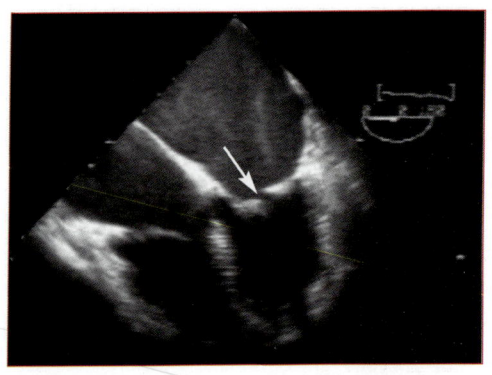

Figure 3. Mitral stenosis with left atrial dilatation. This figure shows a thickened mital valve arrow. The spontaneous contrast is a good illustration of the thrombogenicity of the blood in the left atrium. This is believed to be the first step before the formation of thrombi, which then result in emboli.

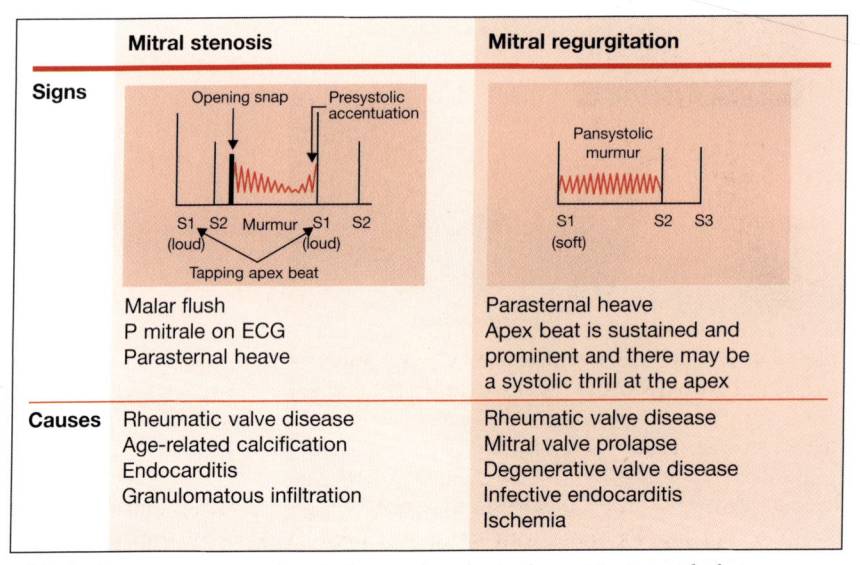

	Mitral stenosis	Mitral regurgitation
Signs	Opening snap, Presystolic accentuation, S1 (loud), S2, Murmur, S1 (loud), S2, Tapping apex beat	Pansystolic murmur, S1 (soft), S2, S3
	Malar flush P mitrale on ECG Parasternal heave	Parasternal heave Apex beat is sustained and prominent and there may be a systolic thrill at the apex
Causes	Rheumatic valve disease Age-related calcification Endocarditis Granulomatous infiltration	Rheumatic valve disease Mitral valve prolapse Degenerative valve disease Infective endocarditis Ischemia

Table 3. Common murmurs in mitral stenosis and mitral regurgitation with their associated signs and causes.

physical signs are described in **Table 4**. **Figure 4** demonstrates MS in echo, electrocardiography pressure tracing, and a chest x-ray.

Natural history

The disease takes a slow course with progressive acceleration later in life. In developed countries, the lag period from the time of rheumatic fever to the onset of symptoms is 20–40 years, and there is another 10 years before these symptoms

Valve disease

Typical physical signs of mitral stenosis
Irregular pulse of atrial fibrillation
Rise in jugular venous pressure (with coexistent tricuspid regurgitation)
Parasternal heave with right ventricular hypertrophy
Loud first heart sound
Tapping apex beat (manifestation of a loud first heart sound)
Opening snap, which disappears as the leaflets become rigid
Classic late diastolic murmur with presystolic accentuation (the longer the murmur, the more severe the lesion)

Table 4. The typical physical signs of mitral stenosis.

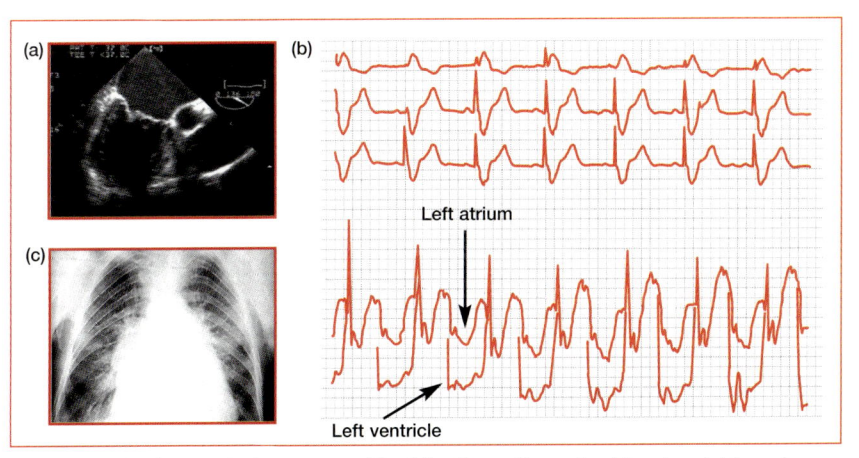

Figure 4. Mitral stenosis demonstrated by (**a**) echocardiography (showing thickened leaflets that no longer open), (**b**) electrocardiography pressure tracing in the left atrium versus left ventricle demonstrating the gradient between the two cavities (and therefore mitral stenosis), and (**c**) chest x-ray.

become disabling. The 10-year survival rate is high for asymptomatic patients (>80%), but low for those with symptoms (0%–15%). Asymptomatic patients with mild MS (MV area >1.5 cm^2) require no further evaluation and do not need to be followed up more than annually.

Percutaneous and surgical therapy
Decisions on therapy are made by joint consideration of symptoms and MV morphology (including hemodynamics and pulmonary artery pressure). Therapeutic options include MV repair (open/closed commissurotomy), MV replacement, and percutaneous valvotomy.

Current recommendations for surgical therapy	
Percutaneous valvotomy	NYHA class II–IV symptoms, MVA <1.5 cm^2, and no LA thrombus or MR
	Asymptomatic patients, MVA ≤1.5 cm^2, pulmonary hypertension (>50 mm Hg), and no LA thrombus or MR
	NYHA class III–IV symptoms, MVA ≤1.5 cm^2, and at high surgical risk
MV repair	NYHA class III–IV symptoms, MVA ≤1.5 cm^2, and one of the following: • percutaneous valvotomy is not available • LA thrombus is resistant to anticoagulation • an intraoperative decision on repair versus replacement will be made
MV replacement	NYHA class I–II symptoms, MVA ≤1 cm^2, and severe pulmonary hypertension (>60 mm Hg)
	NYHA class III–IV symptoms, MVA ≤1.5 cm^2, and not suitable for repair or valvotomy (calcification, fibrosis, subvalvular fusion)

Table 5. Current recommendations for surgical therapy. LA: left atrium; MR: mitral regurgitation; MV: mitral valve; MVA: mitral valve area; NYHA: New York Heart Association.

Both repair and percutaneous valvotomy acutely result in a doubling of the valve area and a 60% reduction in transmitral gradient. However, open commissurotomy and percutaneous valvotomy produce better long-term hemodynamic results. The current recommendations for percutaneous and surgical therapy are outlined in **Table 5**.

Medical therapy
Prophylaxis against rheumatic fever and endocarditis should be considered for all patients with MS. Agents with negative chronotropic properties, such as β-blockers or calcium-channel blockers, may benefit those in sinus rhythm with symptoms relating to exertional tachycardia.

Atrial fibrillation
AF develops in 40% of patients with symptomatic MS and should be treated according to standard protocols (see Chapter 8, Arrhythmia). The value of anticoagulation therapy for those with AF and those with a prior embolic event with or without AF is clear. However, there is no evidence that oral anticoagulation is beneficial in those with MS who have neither AF nor a prior embolic event. The frequency of embolic events does not seem to be related to the severity of MS, the size of the LA, or the presence of symptoms. There is some controversy over

Valve disease

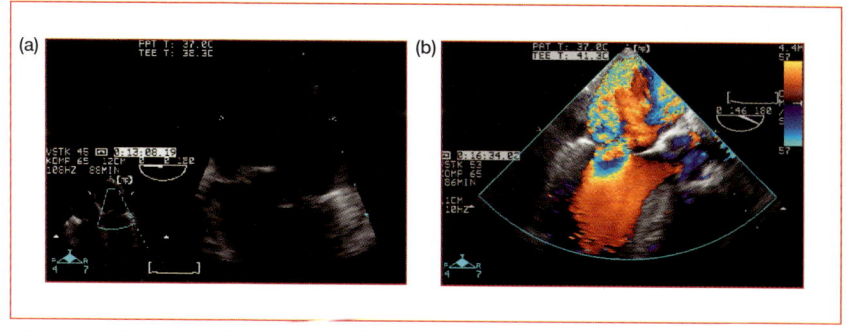

Figure 5. (a) Transesophageal echocardiography showing a tear in the papillary muscle (the most common cause of acute mitral regurgitation). (b) The same scene with a color jet from the left ventricle into the left atrium, demonstrating "blood flow" in the wrong direction.

whether percutaneous mitral valvotomy should be performed in patients with new-onset AF and moderate or severe MS who are otherwise asymptomatic.

Mitral regurgitation

Acute mitral regurgitation

In acute severe mitral regurgitation (MR), the hemodynamic changes are not tolerated and the result is generally acute decompensation. Without time for compensatory LV and LA dilatation, the increase in ventricular preload leads to a decreased stroke volume and pulmonary congestion. However, examination findings may not be typical:

- there may be no hyperdynamic apex beat
- the systolic murmur may be short
- there may be a fourth heart sound

The most common cause of acute MR is papillary muscle rupture secondary to myocardial infarction (MI) (see **Figure 5**). In this situation, the principal differential diagnosis is ventricular septal defect and an echo is required to differentiate between the two. Ventricular septal defect is more likely with:

- right-sided radiation of murmur
- raised jugular venous pressure (JVP)
- anterior MI (inferior MI is more likely to cause acute MR)

The goal of medical therapy in acute severe MR is to diminish regurgitation, increase stroke volume, and reduce pulmonary congestion. As such, nitroprusside alone or in combination with dobutamine (if blood pressure is low) can be

Chapter 9

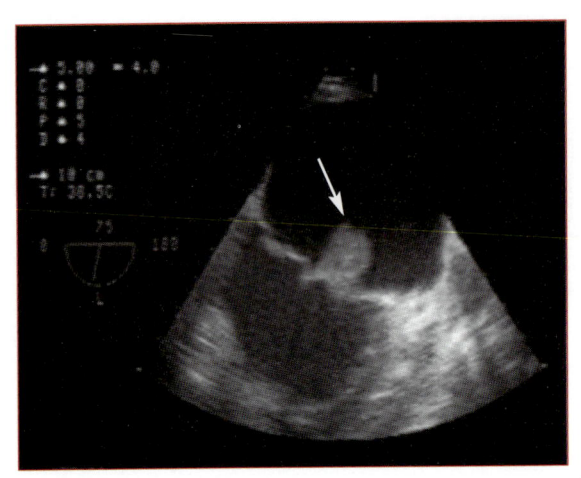

Figure 6. Echocardiogram showing a vegetation on the mitral valve (arrow).

Clinical signs of chronic mitral regurgitation
Prominent and sustained apex beat
Systolic thrill at the apex
Left parasternal heave – resulting from left atrium expansion, rather than right ventricular hypertrophy
Soft first heart sound
Pansystolic murmur at the apex that radiates into the axilla
Third heart sound that is high pitched due to high early diastolic filling velocities

Table 6. The clinical signs of chronic mitral regurgitation.

effective. Intra-aortic balloon pumping can also help to achieve these goals. In many cases, emergency surgery is warranted. If so, prior transesophageal echo helps to characterize the anatomy and severity of the lesion. Cardiac catheterization should be performed if the patient is at high risk for CAD.

Chronic mitral regurgitation
Causes

- Degenerative MV disease is common in the elderly. The valve leaflets are thickened, redundant, increased in area, and they prolapse into the LA in systole. The chordae may become elongated, thinned, and tortuous – predisposing to rupture.

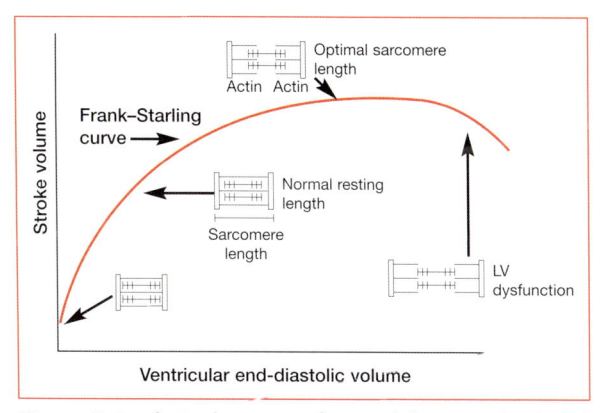

Figure 7. Frank–Starling curve showing left ventricular (LV) dysfunction.

- Infective endocarditis is a major cause of chronic MR. Vegetations developing on the cusp vary from small nodules along the line of apposition to large friable masses of up to 10 mm or more (see **Figure 6**). "Jet" lesions on the anterior cusp of the MV can also occur in association with aortic valve endocarditis.
- Ischemia.

Clinical signs

The clinical signs of chronic MR are outlined in **Table 6**. With severe MR, the regurgitant murmur is usually short and stops at the same time as aortic valve closure. Occasionally, the murmur can hardly be heard due to early equalization of atrioventricular pressures. The signs and causes of MR are outlined in **Table 3**.

Natural history

In chronic MR, the increased preload and decreased afterload of the LV (caused by ejection of some of the stroke volume into the LA) are compensated for by LV and LA dilatation, and the total stroke volume is increased (the EF is also maintained). This compensated phase of chronic MR may last for years. Eventually, however, the volume overload causes sufficient dilatation to push the LV onto the downward portion of the Frank–Starling curve and dysfunction results (see **Figure 7**). Importantly, the loading conditions mean that this dysfunction might not be reflected in an abnormal EF (the EF in a patient with MR and normal LV function is >60%).

Asymptomatic patients with mild MR and no evidence of LV dilatation or dysfunction can be followed on a yearly basis and undergo echo less frequently than that. Asymptomatic patients with moderate MR should have an echo annually. Asymptomatic patients with severe MR should be followed up every

6–12 months and undergo echo to detect silent LV dysfunction. Exercise testing is useful to document changes in exercise tolerance.

The timing of surgery is determined by the EF, LV end systolic dimension (LVESD), the presence of AF, and symptoms. It is indicated for those with:

- class II–IV symptoms, EF >60%, LVESD <45 mm
- EF 30%–60%, LVESD 45–55 mm (regardless of symptoms)
- asymptomatic patients with AF and normal EF
- symptomatic patients with normal EF and pulmonary hypertension (>50 mm Hg)
- asymptomatic patients with EF 50%–60% and LVESD <45 mm, or EF >60% and LVESD 45–55 mm
- patients with EF <30% and/or LVESD >55 mm in whom the chordae tendineae are likely to be intact (ie, no previous MI in that territory)

The operation of choice is MV repair. In many patients, however, replacement of the valve together with removal of part or all of the MV apparatus (chordae) is required. The repair procedure leads to better postoperative LV function and survival.

There is no generally accepted medical therapy for chronic MR. Although vasodilators might seem a sensible choice, in fact, in compensated chronic MR the afterload is decreased (since the LV has two routes of ejection); as such, drugs that reduce the afterload further are unlikely to be beneficial.

Chronic MR can also occur due to a primary ischemic cause, relating either to LV dysfunction or to chordal ischemia – revascularization or stenting can eliminate the episodes.

Functional mitral regurgitation
The normal function of the MV depends on the cusps, ring, and subvalvular apparatus, including papillary muscle fibers and the circumferential muscle layer supporting the mitral ring. Each of these components plays a significant role in maintaining the competence of the valve. With papillary muscle dysfunction due to ischemia or other causes of ventricular disease, cusp closure is not complete, leading to some degree of regurgitation. This can even occur, for example, in athletic hypertrophy. This is usually mild, but can be significant in rare cases. In such conditions, the heart rate is usually fast and the duration of MR long enough to compromise filling time and hence cardiac output. Although functional in origin, it can be hemodynamically significant.

Valve disease

> **ALFRED DE MUSSET**
> "La bouche garde le silence,
> Pour écouter parler le coeur."[a]
> Alfred de Musset (1810–1857), *La Nuit de Mai*
>
> The French romantic poet and playwright, Alfred de Musset (1810–1857), was famous for both his creative brain and his pathological heart. His most inspiring work was prompted by the ending of a love affair he had with George Sand (a French romantic writer who later had a 10-year relationship with Chopin). During a visit to Venice in 1834, both Sand and he became very unwell. Such was the quality of care and attention lavished on them by their physician that Sand fell in love with this man and de Musset returned to France alone (where he penned some of his best work). He spent the last 2 years of his life housebound, his heart broken by the combined effects of lost love, aortic regurgitation, and alcohol-related cardiomyopathy. The nodding of his head in time with his heartbeat, the classic eponymous sign of aortic regurgitation, was described by his brother in a biography. When told of it, de Musset apparently placed his thumb and forefinger on his neck and his head stopped bobbing.
> [a]The mouth keeps silent to hear the heart speak.

Mitral valve prolapse

MV prolapse (MVP) is the single most common valvular abnormality. It affects 2%–6% of the population and is defined as a backward movement of one or both leaflets of the MV (usually the anterior) into the LA during (ventricular) systole. In most cases it is associated with trivial MR. However, as a result of its prevalence, it is also the most common single cause of significant MR. Although MVP does not alter life expectancy, all of the above complications of MR can occur. Sudden death, often reported as an association with MVP, is rare (<2% on long-term follow-up).

Classic findings on auscultation are a mid systolic click followed by a late systolic murmur. The click is thought to be caused by a tensing of the MV apparatus as the leaflets prolapse into the LA. The murmur is usually high pitched and loudest at the apex. Certain maneuvers can help to secure the diagnosis: standing reduces end diastolic volume (EDV), bringing the click–murmur nearer to the first heart sound; squatting increases EDV (and afterload), moving the click–murmur nearer to the second heart sound.

Patients with these findings should be referred for echo assessment. Interestingly, there is no absolute consensus on criteria for diagnosing MVP on two-dimensional echo. The diagnosis should never be made on one view alone (especially if that is the 4-chamber view). Serial echos are not necessary unless there is a change in the clinical picture.

Management involves reassurance and prophylaxis for endocarditis. Patients who suffer from palpitations should have Holter/event monitoring to make a firm diagnosis. Aspirin is recommended for patients with documented focal neurological events who are in sinus rhythm and have no atrial thrombus. Recurrent transient ischemic attacks or stroke in MVP patients demand long-term warfarin therapy. Ultimately, MV repair may be required, and the indications are as for MR (described above).

Tricuspid valve disease

In comparison with the left side, the right side of the heart is a low-pressure system. Consequently, disorders such as endocarditis, in which high-pressure jets help to "seed" the infective vegetations, occur less frequently. The notable exception is in intravenous drug abusers, where right-sided endocarditis is more common. Perhaps the most common cause of tricuspid valve incompetence, however, is elevated right ventricular (RV) pressure, secondary to pulmonary hypertension, MS, pulmonary stenosis, dilated cardiomyopathy, or RV failure. In addition, rheumatic heart disease can affect the tricuspid valve and tends to produce a combination of tricuspid stenosis and regurgitation – the overriding symptoms are those of regurgitation. Ebstein's anomaly is a congenital disorder affecting the tricuspid valve (see Chapter 14, Adult congenital heart disease).

Clinical signs
Physical examination is key to the diagnosis of tricuspid regurgitation. Typical signs are:

- gross fluid retention
- significant peripheral edema
- ascites that may result in nausea
- raised JVP with a prominent systolic wave and sharp Y descent
- parasternal heave and loud P2, suggesting pulmonary hypertension as a cause
- an enlarged, tender, pulsatile liver and, occasionally, mild jaundice
- a pansystolic murmur at the left lower sternal edge that is increased by inspiration

Management
Severe tricuspid regurgitation resulting from any cause is associated with a poor long-term outcome due to RV dysfunction and systemic venous congestion. The timing of surgery and the most suitable operation remain controversial, although chordal reconstruction and annuloplasty have become established in recent years.

Annuloplasty involves the use of a prosthetic ring to support the endogenous dilated annulus. Valve replacement is also possible.

Medical management treats fluid retention and AF. Standard protocols are used, although high doses and combination diuretics are often required.

Pulmonary valve disease

Pulmonary regurgitation is caused by pulmonary hypertension and annular dilatation resulting from various causes of left-sided heart disease (as well as primary pulmonary hypertension). An early diastolic murmur (Graham Steell murmur) is heard over the pulmonary area and should be distinguished from that of AR.

Antibiotic prophylaxis is only required if the cause is rheumatic. Most pulmonary valve disease does not need treatment. However, valve replacement can be carried out in cases of intractable right heart failure.

Valve disease in pregnancy

In pregnancy, there is a 50% increase in circulating blood volume. The cardiac output peaks between the second and third trimesters, predominantly due to an increase in stroke volume, although the heart rate also increases by up to 20%. Total peripheral resistance falls disproportionately, reducing the diastolic blood pressure and widening the pulse pressure. Occasionally, in the supine position the inferior vena cava can be compressed by a gravid uterus, leading to an abrupt decrease in venous return. This can result in light headedness, but quickly resolves on changing position. The increased blood volume and cardiac output can accentuate stenotic murmurs, while the lowered peripheral resistance can actually reduce regurgitant murmurs. In general, echo demonstrates a degree of "physiological" chamber enlargement that, in a significant minority of women, may be associated with functional MR.

In some conditions (eg, cyanotic heart disease, Eisenmenger syndrome, and severe pulmonary hypertension), the changes resulting from pregnancy greatly increase risk and most cardiologists would counsel against pregnancy. The following are also associated with increased risk, either to the mother or fetus:

- severe AS
- MR/AR with class III–IV symptoms
- MS with class II–IV symptoms
- pulmonary pressures >75% of systemic
- EF <40%
- mechanical prosthetic valves requiring anticoagulation
- AR in Marfan's syndrome

Although risk is increased, many patients with valvular abnormalities can be managed through pregnancy with conservative medical measures aimed at optimizing intravascular volume.

Mitral stenosis
Penicillin prophylaxis should be continued in pregnant women with MS. The cautious use of diuretics and β-blockers in those with mild to moderate disease can prevent tachycardia and optimize diastolic filling. For women with severe disease, a percutaneous balloon valvotomy prior to conception should be considered. Those who develop class III–IV symptoms during pregnancy should also undergo valvotomy. This can be achieved with very limited fluoroscopy or appropriate shielding.

Mitral regurgitation
The usual cause of MR is MVP; this rarely requires treatment.

Aortic stenosis
The most likely cause of AS in a woman of childbearing age is congenital bicuspid disease. Mild to moderate obstruction can be managed conservatively throughout pregnancy, whereas those with severe disease (eg, gradient >50 mm Hg, LV function likely to be normal) should be advised to delay conception until treatment is obtained.

Aortic regurgitation
AR can usually be managed medically with a combination of diuretics and vasodilator therapy. As with MR, surgery should be contemplated during pregnancy for the control of class III–IV symptoms.

Anticoagulation in pregnancy
Warfarin crosses the placenta and has been associated with an increased incidence of spontaneous abortion, fetal deformity, prematurity, and stillbirth. The incidence is probably around 5%–10%. In contrast, heparin does not cross the placenta and is generally safer. However, it is associated with a higher degree of thromboembolic complications. The evidence base for decision making is not good, and the decision should be made in partnership with the patient after explaining the risks involved. Most change from warfarin to heparin at week 36 in anticipation of labor.

Further reading

Guidelines for the management of patients with valvular heart disease. Executive summary: a report of the American College of Cardiology/American Heart Association Task Force on Practice Guidelines (Committee on Management of Patients with Valvular Heart Disease). *Circulation* 1998;98:1949–84.

Phoon CK. Estimation of pressure gradients by auscultations: an innovative and accurate physical examination technique. *Am Heart J* 2001;141:500–6.

Shry EA, Smithers MA, Mascette AM. Auscultation versus echocardiography in a healthy population with precordial murmur. *Am J Cardiol* 2001;87:1428–30.

Chapter 10

Infective endocarditis

Background

Endocarditis was first described by William Osler in 1885. It is an inflammatory process that affects the endocardium and may have an infective or noninfective (eg, systemic lupus erythematosus) origin. It is uncommon in the western world (22 cases per million), but more prevalent in developing countries.

Diagnosis

Symptoms
Endocarditis is rarely an obvious diagnosis for a generalist. It may present with a wide variety of clinical signs, some subtle; the diagnosis may be difficult or the signs misleading, and there is a wide differential diagnosis to consider. However, there is a wealth of clinical signs to look for.

Constitutional symptoms
Endocarditis should be considered in patients with vague or generalized constitutional symptoms such as fever, rigors, night sweats, anorexia, weight loss, or arthralgia.

Cardiac signs
The presence of a new murmur is very significant, as is a change in the nature of an existing murmur (a regurgitant murmur may disappear on worsening). Myocardial involvement or valvular dysfunction may both contribute to left ventricular failure.

Skin lesions
Endocarditis is indicated by:
- Osler's nodes – tender lesions found on finger pulps and thenar/hypothenar eminences (see **Figure 1**)
- Janeway lesions – transient, nontender macular papules on palms or soles
- splinter hemorrhages
- petechiae (embolic or vasculitic)
- clubbing – in long-standing disease

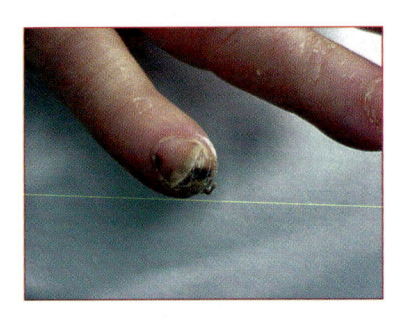

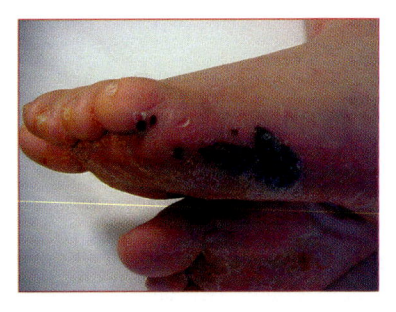

Figure 1. Osler's nodes on a finger and foot.

Eyes
Roth spots (boat-shaped hemorrhages with pale centers, in retina) and conjunctival splinter hemorrhages may be found.

Splenomegaly
Splenic infarction may occur as a result of emboli. In this case, splenic palpation may be painful and tender, and a rub may be heard.

Neurological
An acute confusional state is common in patients with infective endocarditis (IE). Cerebral emboli, which usually affect the middle cerebral artery, result in hemiplegia and sensory dysfunction. Mycotic aneurysms also affect the middle cerebral artery, where rupture may cause a subarachnoid hematoma. Mycotic aneurysms can occur several years after endocarditis has been treated.

Renal
Infarction causes loin pain and hematuria. Immune complex deposition may result in glomerulonephritis.

OSLER'S NODES
William Osler, 1909, on the eponymous Osler's nodes: "One of the most interesting features of [endocarditis] and one to which very little attention has been paid is the occurrence of ephemeral spots of a painful nodular erythema, chiefly in the skin of the hands and feet, the nodosités cutanées éphémerès of the French... The commonest situation is near the tip of the finger, which may be slightly swollen."

If any of these signs occur together with a fever, the patient should be urgently referred to a cardiologist for blood cultures and echocardiography – the level of risk will determine whether this is transesophageal echo (TEE) or transthoracic echo. Blind treatment with antibiotics should not be undertaken since it will delay diagnosis and identification of the causal organism. Antibiotics should not be initiated before three sets of blood cultures have been taken.

Formal diagnosis

The Duke diagnostic classification for IE divides signs and symptoms into major and minor criteria (see **Table 1**). IE is diagnosed if patients have:

- two major criteria; or
- one major and three minor criteria; or
- five minor criteria

These criteria are associated with a 99% specificity for diagnosis in follow-up studies. It has been proposed that the minor criteria be extended to include erythrocyte sedimentation rate (ESR) or C-reactive protein (CRP), splenomegaly, microscopic hematuria, and newly diagnosed clubbing. This adjustment increases diagnostic sensitivity by 10%.

Intravenous drug abuse

Right-sided endocarditis is common in intravenous drug abusers (IVDAs) because of nonsterile injection into the venous system. The presentation tends to differ from that of classic IE, in that these patients are more likely to develop pneumonia or septic pulmonary emboli than the characteristic signs mentioned above (which result from left-sided embolization). In addition, predominant right-sided failure is more common (look for significantly raised jugular venous pressure and gross peripheral edema). The tricuspid valve is most commonly affected (50%), whereas involvement of the mitral and aortic valves is less common (20% each). The involvement of multiple valves is common. Pulmonary valve endocarditis is rare.

Etiology

IE has a large number of causative organisms.

Streptococci

These account for 50%–80% of IE cases. *Streptococcus viridans* (eg, *S. anguis*, *S. milleri*, *S. mutans*, *S. mitior*) make up the normal bacterial flora of the pharynx and upper respiratory tract. Tonsillectomy, dental extraction, and dental cleaning can result in bacteremia and lead to infection.

The Duke criteria for the diagnosis of IE

Major criteria

1. Positive blood culture for IE

A. Typical micro-organism consistent with IE from two separate blood cultures, as noted below:
- viridans streptococci, *Streptococcus bovis*[a], or HACEK group; or
- community-acquired *Staphylococcus aureus* or enterococci, in the absence of a primary focus; or

B. Micro-organisms consistent with IE from persistently positive blood cultures defined as:
- two or more positive cultures of blood samples drawn >12 hours apart
- all of three or a majority of four or more separate cultures of blood (with first and last sample drawn ≥1 hour apart)

2. Evidence of endocardial involvement

A. Positive echocardiogram for IE defined as:
- oscillating intracardiac mass on valve or supporting structures, in the path of regurgitant jets, or on implanted material in the absence of an alternative anatomic explanation; or
- abscess; or
- new partial dehiscence of prosthetic valve; or

B. New valvular regurgitation (worsening or changing of pre-existing murmur not sufficient)

Minor criteria

1. Predisposition: predisposing heart condition or intravenous drug use
2. Fever: temperature ≥38.0°C
3. Vascular phenomena: major arterial emboli, septic pulmonary infarcts, mycotic aneurysm, intracranial hemorrhage, conjunctival hemorrhages, and Janeway lesions
4. Immunologic phenomena: glomerulonephritis, Osler's nodes, Roth spots, and rheumatoid factor
5. Microbiological evidence: positive blood culture, but does not meet a major criterion as noted above[b] or serological evidence of active infection with an organism consistent with IE
6. Echocardiography findings: consistent with IE, but do not meet a major criterion as noted above

Table 1. Definitions of terms used in the Duke criteria for the diagnosis of infective endocarditis (IE). HACEK: *Haemophilus parainfluenza, Haemophilus aphrophilus, Actinobacillus (Haemophilus) actinomycetemcomitans, Cardiobacterium hominis, Eikenella* species, and *Kingella* species. [a]Includes nutritionally variant strains (*Abiotrophia* species); [b]excludes single positive cultures for coagulase-negative staphylococci and organisms that do not cause endocarditis. Reproduced with permission from Excerpta Medica (Durack DT, Lukes AS, Bright DK. New criteria for diagnosis of infective endocarditis: utilization of specific echocardiographic findings. Duke Endocarditis Service. *Am J Med* 1994;96:200–9). ©1994 Excerpta Medica.

> **WILLIAM OSLER, 1919:**
> **"Observe, record, tabulate, communicate. Use your five senses."**
> Sir William Osler (1849–1919) is one of the most admired and honored physicians in the history of medicine. He exerted a truly global influence through professorships (McGill, Johns Hopkins, and Oxford), his textbook The Principles and Practice of Medicine, and other clinical and philosophical writings. This influence is apparent not least in the sheer number of conditions that bear his name: Osler–Weber–Rendu syndrome (hereditary hemorrhagic telangiectasia), Osler's nodes, Osler–Libman disease (subacute bacterial endocarditis), and Osler–Libman–Sacks syndrome (systemic lupus erythematosus with endocarditis) are simply a few. But it was perhaps his overwhelming humanism and his dedication to patient-centered learning that marked him out as truly great (he once ran after an alcoholic beggar to whom he'd just given coins and added his own overcoat to the donation, saying: "You may drink yourself to death, and undoubtedly will, but I cannot let you freeze to death"). The combination of profound caring, a prolific output of creative writing and ideas, and a lifelong penchant for elaborate practical jokes has made him one of the most memorable physicians of the 20th century.

Staphylococci

Staphylococcus aureus and *Staphylococcus epidermidis* account for 20%–30% of subacute cases of IE and 50% of the acute forms. The presence of central venous catheters (feeding lines or temporary pacing lines) increases susceptibility. Acute *S. aureus* infection of previously normal valves has a mortality rate of 3%. This is the most common situation in IVDAs. Coagulase-negative staphylococci cause 30%–50% of prosthetic valve endocarditis.

Enterococci

Enterococci account for 5%–15% of IE cases. Enterococcal organisms, which include *Streptococcus faecalis*, have low infectivity.

HACEK organisms

The HACEK group of organisms – *Haemophilus parainfluenza*, *Haemophilus aphrophilus*, *Actinobacillus* (*Haemophilus*) *actinomycetemcomitans*, *Cardiobacterium hominis*, the *Eikenella* species, and the *Kingella* species – also commonly cause IE and can be difficult to diagnose. Their identification may require samples to be taken in special media.

IE is also caused by other, less common organisms. *Candida*, *Aspergillus*, *Histoplasma*, and *Brucella* infections are rare, but are found, in particular, in IVDAs, alcoholics, and patients with prosthetic heart valves. *Coxiella burnetii* (the causative agent of Q fever) can also cause a subacute infection.

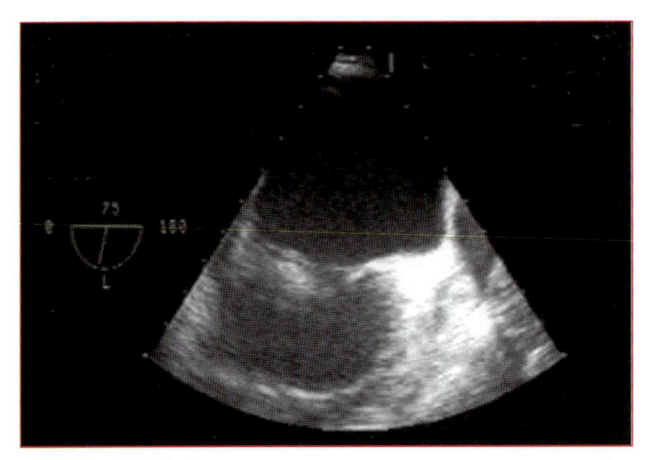

Figure 2. Mitral valve vegetation.

Pathogenesis

Endocarditis infection occurs along the edges of the heart valves. The lesions, called vegetations, are masses composed of fibrin, platelets, and infecting organisms, held together by agglutinating antibodies produced by the bacteria. As inflammation continues, ulceration may result in erosion or perforation of the valve cusps, leading to valvular incompetence, damage to the conduction pathway (if in the septal area), or rupture of a sinus of Valsalva (if in the aortic area).

Although endocarditis can affect native and prosthetic valves, infection seldom affects a previously normal heart – the majority (60%) of IE patients have a predisposing cardiac condition. Vegetations usually affect the left side of the heart, with the most common underlying lesions being mitral valve prolapse and degenerative mitral and aortic regurgitation (see **Figure 2**).

Rheumatic disease is a risk factor for the development of endocarditis. Other predisposing cardiac lesions include hypertrophic cardiomyopathy with associated mitral reflux, subaortic stenosis, and ventricular aneurysm. There are also congenital lesions that predispose adults to endocarditis: these include ventricular septal defect (VSD), bicuspid aortic valve, and coarctation of the aorta.

Vegetations occur when a high-pressure jet enters a low-pressure cavity through a narrow orifice. This explains why endocarditis complicates a small VSD, but is not associated with a large VSD, mitral stenosis, or an atrial septal defect. In the presence of a VSD, vegetations can be found on the right ventricular side of the VSD, on the tricuspid valve, or where the jet impinges on the right ventricular wall. Vegetations found in coarctation usually occur distal to the obstruction.

Finally, in children, cyanotic heart disease is still the most common cause of endocarditis, and the risk does not diminish after surgical repair as prostheses carry their own risk.

Prosthetic valve endocarditis
A special subset of endocarditis is that affecting prosthetic valves. This is traditionally divided into early onset (within 60 days of surgery) or late onset. Early onset usually results from perioperative valve contamination with staphylococci, whereas the etiology of late prosthetic valve endocarditis resembles native valve infection, usually due to streptococci.

Refer with confidence
As mentioned above, IE can be a difficult diagnosis to make, and the key for the generalist is to always be aware of it as a differential. Fever and arthralgia are very common complaints, but if there is any suggestion that they are not due to a simple viral illness (eg, by the presence of a particularly high temperature or other clinical signs [see above]) then the patient should be referred for blood cultures and an echo. If fever and a changing murmur coexist then urgent referral is warranted, although, even here, it can be useful to take blood cultures and a bottle for serology (for the diagnosis of culture-negative endocarditis) yourself.

Specialist management
Investigations
Blood cultures
Blood cultures are the primary investigation in the diagnosis of IE and yield the causative micro-organism in up to 95% of cases. A failure to do so can be due to prior antibiotic treatment, the presence of fastidious organisms (eg, belonging to the HACEK group), or unusual organisms such as *Candida*, *Chlamydia*, or *Brucella*. Most importantly, blood has to be drawn before antibiotic treatment is initiated, at three different time points over a minimum of 1 hour. At each time point, blood should be taken from a different site of the patient's body – but not from central lines – and each sample is placed into a pair of blood culture bottles that cultivate aerobic and anaerobic bacteria separately.

If immediate antibiotic treatment is warranted, this can be initiated right after completion of blood culturing, once microbiology tests have identified a specific organism and the antibiotic therapy has been modified accordingly. Antibiotic therapy can have an enormous impact on the patient's prognosis; therefore, all efforts have to be made to collect and culture specimens as carefully as possible. This ensures the correct identification of the causative micro-organisms, and ultimately the correct use of antibiotics.

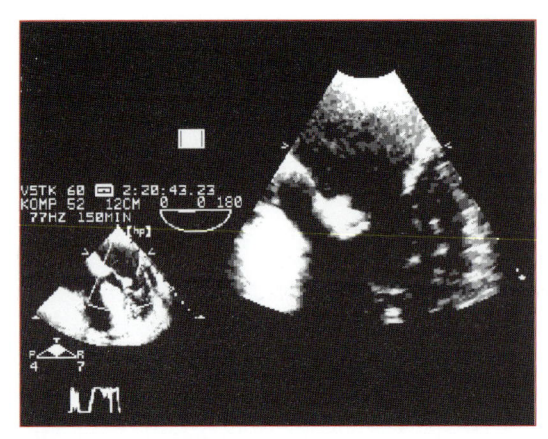

Figure 3. Transesophageal echo for 1 mm lesions.

Echocardiography
This is the key investigation as it can assess underlying cardiac function as well as demonstrate vegetations. Chamber size, pre-existing rheumatic disease, and valve apparatus can be examined and the degree of valve incompetence assessed. Transthoracic two-dimensional echo can detect vegetations above 2 mm in diameter, whereas TEE has greater precision in detection of lesions (1–1.5 mm), with a sensitivity and specificity of over 90% (see **Figure 3**). Detection of prosthetic endocarditis is more sensitive with TEE.

Other investigations
Other investigations include the following:

- blood count – normochromic normocytic anemia is usual, while neutrophil leucocytosis is common
- ESR – this may be raised
- renal and liver function test – levels of creatinine may be raised; levels of liver enzymes may be raised in a hepatocellular (nonobstructive) pattern
- CRP – increases acutely in bacterial infection
- urine microscopy – microscopic hematuria is common in early disease
- culture – culture any skin lesion, drip site, or other focus of infection
- electrocardiography (ECG) – ECG regularly (daily if aortic or septal root abscess is suspected)

Treatment
Antibiotics
If, following blood cultures, the diagnosis is secure, high-dose IV antibiotics should be started immediately. It is becoming increasingly common to insert a

tunneled central line to facilitate several weeks of IV treatment without the need for repeated cannulation – with the pain and attendant risk of secondary infection that this incurs.

Native valve endocarditis with a subacute onset is most likely to be caused by *S. viridans* or an enterococcal species. Treatment involves IV penicillin (2.4 g, 4 hourly) for up to 4 weeks, with gentamicin (1 mg/kg, 12 hourly) for 2 weeks. If the onset is acute, staphylococci need to be covered and treatment should include IV cloxacillin (flucloxacillin) (3 g, 6 hourly, in place of penicillin) with oral fusidic acid.

If the patient is allergic to penicillin, other possibilities are vancomycin (1 g twice daily) or teicoplanin (400 mg twice daily for 3 days, then 400 mg daily). Plasma levels of gentamicin and vancomycin need to be monitored every 48–72 hours.

Empirical treatment of endocarditis affecting prosthetic valves should cover streptococci, enterococci, staphylococci (including methicillin-resistant *S. aureus*), and Gram-negative organisms. Vancomycin or teicoplanin with gentamicin have good synergistic cover. In drug abusers, treatment for endocarditis should include cover for *S. aureus* and Gram-negative bacilli (eg, cloxacillin and pipercillin).

In the treatment of rarer causes of endocarditis, *Coxiella* may require doxycycline with cotrimoxazole or rifampicin. *Candida* and *Aspergillus* may respond to medical therapy (5-fluorouracil and amphotericin B, respectively), but, generally, all three of these infections respond poorly to medical therapy alone and require surgical intervention.

In the treatment of IE, from any source, fever may still be present 2 weeks after starting the appropriate treatment, even with drug-sensitive organisms. This could be due to the presence of an underlying large vegetation or abscess. If fever persists, the sensitivity of the infecting organism should be checked and drug levels monitored. Repeat echo should be performed to exclude increasing vegetation size or abscess formation. If, despite these measures, the fever remains, the possibility of antibiotic resistance should be considered and a further synergistic antimicrobial treatment may be required. A second site for fever should always be excluded.

Surgical intervention
Surgical intervention may be required in patients with persistent fever that is resistant to medical therapy. Surgery is also indicated in the following conditions:

- valve obstruction
- prosthetic-valve endocarditis caused by *S. aureus* or resistant organisms
- aortic or mitral regurgitation not responding to medical therapy
- paravalvular abscess
- development of an aneurysm of a sinus of Valsalva
- fungal endocarditis
- multiple embolic episodes
- progressive heart failure secondary to severe valve destruction
- oscillating vegetation of >1 cm

Surgery may involve not only valve replacement, but also aortic root replacement for aortic root abscesses. After the relevant surgical procedure, a full course of antibiotic eradication therapy should be administered.

Prognosis

With effective treatment, patients with IE have a 70% survival rate. The prognosis is worse if there is no identifiable organism or if there is a resistant organism. Fungal infections are associated with increased mortality, as is prosthetic valve endocarditis. Overall death rates are 20% for native valve endocarditis, 30% for staphylococcal infections, and 20%–30% for late prosthetic valve infection, despite full medical and surgical treatment. The most common cause of death is intractable heart failure.

Prophylaxis

All patients at risk for IE should receive antibiotic cover for invasive procedures (see **Tables 2** and **3**, overleaf). Spontaneous bacteremia is also common as a result of poor dental hygiene, and susceptible patients need to be made aware of this.

Infective endocarditis

Situation	Agent[a]	Regimen
Standard general prophylaxis	Amoxicillin	Adults: 2 g; children: 50 mg/kg orally 1 hour before procedure
Unable to take oral medication	Ampicillin	Adults: 2 g IM or IV; children: 50 mg/kg IM or IV within 30 minutes before procedure
Allergic to penicillin	Clindamycin	Adults: 600 mg; children: 20 mg/kg orally 1 hour before procedure
	Cephalexin[b], cefadroxil[b]	Adults: 2 g; children; 50 mg/kg orally 1 hour before procedure
	Azithromycin, clarithromycin	Adults: 500 mg; children: 15 mg/kg orally 1 hour before procedure
Allergic to penicillin and unable to take oral medications	Clindamycin	Adults: 600 mg; children: 20 mg/kg IV within 30 minutes before procedure
	Cefazolin[b]	Adults: 1 g; children: 25 mg/kg IM or IV within 30 minutes before procedure

Table 2. Prophylactic regimens for dental, oral, respiratory tract, or esophageal procedures. IM: intramuscularly; IV: intravenously. [a]Total children's dose should not exceed adult dose; [b]cephalosporins should not be used in individuals with immediate-type hypersensitivity reaction (urticaria, angioedema, or anaphylaxis) to penicillins. Reproduced with permission from Lippincott Williams & Wilkins (Dajani AS, Taubert KA, Wilson W et al. Prevention of Bacterial Endocarditis: Recommendations by the American Heart Association. *Circulation* 1997;96:358–66).

Situation	Agents[a]	Regimen[b]
High-risk patients	Ampicillin + gentamicin	Adults: ampicillin 2 g IM or IV plus gentamicin 1.5 mg/kg (not to exceed 120 mg) within 30 minutes of starting the procedure; 6 hours later, ampicillin 1 g IM/IV or amoxicillin 1 g orally
		Children: ampicillin 50 mg/kg IM or IV (not to exceed 2 g) + gentamicin 1.5 mg/kg within 30 minutes of starting the procedure; 6 hours later, ampicillin 25 mg/kg IM/IV or amoxicillin 25 mg/kg orally
High-risk patients allergic to ampicillin/ amoxicillin	Vancomycin + gentamicin	Adults: vancomycin 1 g IV over 1–2 hours + gentamicin 1.5 mg/kg IV/IM (not to exceed 120 mg); complete injection/infusion within 30 minutes of starting the procedure
		Children: vancomycin 20 mg/kg IV over 1–2 hours + gentamicin 1.5 mg/kg IV/IM; complete injection/infusion within 30 minutes of starting the procedure
Moderate-risk patients	Amoxicillin or ampicillin	Adults: amoxicillin 2 g orally 1 hour before procedure, or ampicillin 2 g IM/IV within 30 minutes of starting the procedure
		Children: amoxicillin 50 mg/kg orally 1 hour before procedure, or ampicillin 50 mg/kg IM/IV within 30 minutes of starting the procedure
Moderate-risk patients allergic to ampicillin/amoxicillin	Vancomycin	Adults: vancomycin 1 g IV over 1–2 hours; complete infusion within 30 minutes of starting the procedure
		Children: vancomycin 20 mg/kg IV over 1–2 hours; complete infusion within 30 minutes of starting the procedure

Table 3. Prophylactic regimens for genitourinary/gastrointestinal (excluding esophageal) procedures. IM: intramuscularly; IV: intravenously. [a]Total children's dose should not exceed adult dose; [b]no second dose of vancomycin or gentamicin is recommended. Reproduced with permission from Lippincott Williams & Wilkins (Dajani AS, Taubert KA, Wilson W et al. Prevention of Bacterial Endocarditis: Recommendations by the American Heart Association. *Circulation* 1997;96:358–66).

Further reading

Bayer AS, Bolger AF, Taubert KA et al. Diagnosis and management of IE and its complications. AHA Scientific Statement. *Circulation* 1998;98:2936–48.

Dajani AS, Taubert KA, Wilson W et al. Prevention of Bacterial Endocarditis: Recommendations by the American Heart Association. *Circulation* 1997;96:358–66.

Golden RL. William Osler at 150. *JAMA* 1999;282:2252–8.

Chapter 11

Cardiomyopathy

Hypertrophic cardiomyopathy

With a prevalence of only 0.2%, hypertrophic cardiomyopathy (HCM) is rarely encountered by generalists. Most cases are identified by screening family members of known sufferers – 50% of cases are familial.

Background

HCM is a primary, usually familial disorder of cardiac muscle with complex pathophysiology, significant heterogeneity in its expression, and a diverse clinical course. It is defined as cardiac hypertrophy that cannot be explained by pressure or volume overload, and is probably the most common genetically transmitted heart disease. The clinical course is highly variable; some patients remain asymptomatic throughout life, whereas others die prematurely – either suddenly or from progressive heart failure. HCM is characterized by mutations in the DNA encoding cardiac contractile or energy-related proteins, predominantly the β-myosin heavy chain, α-tropomyosin, and cardiac troponin T (see **Figure 1** and **Table 1**).

Despite dramatic improvements in the knowledge and understanding of HCM, challenges and controversies still exist regarding its diagnosis, etiology, natural history, and management. For example, many HCM patients do not, in fact, have left ventricular hypertrophy (LVH). The shifting understanding of this complex disease can make terminology difficult. However, "hypertrophic cardiomyopathy" is the preferred expression for this condition. This nomenclature avoids the term "idiopathic subaortic stenosis" or inclusion of the word "obstructive", which imply left ventricular outflow tract obstruction (present in only 25% of cases). It also excludes secondary causes of LVH.

The classic features of HCM are asymmetrical LVH with a normal or small left ventricular cavity. However, wall thickness varies considerably. The majority of clearly identified patients have an unmistakably abnormal left ventricular mass. This averages at a septal thickness of 20–22 mm, but can be up to 60 mm (see **Figure 2**). This leaves a significant minority of patients in whom there will be diagnostic ambiguity with respect to cardiac morphology. In fact, the hallmark of the disease is

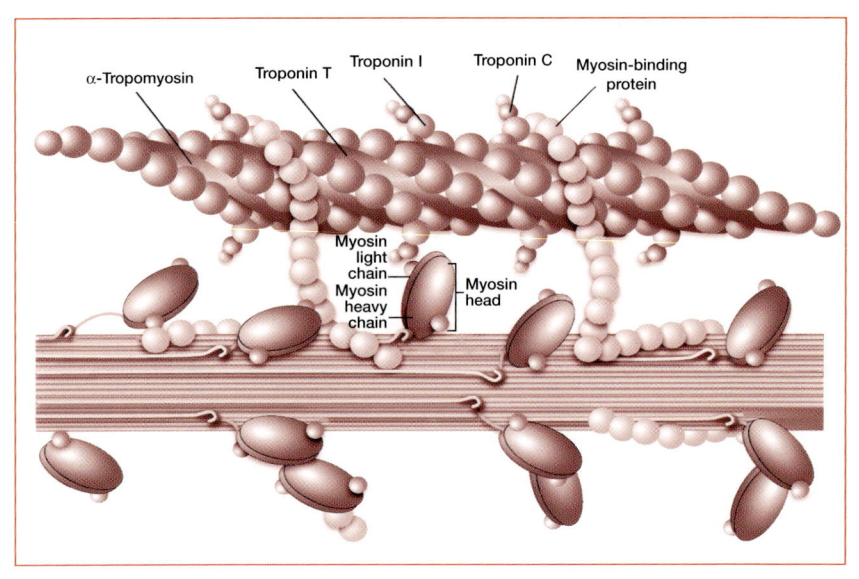

Figure 1. Contractile proteins in the cardiac sarcomere. The top chain represents actin; the bottom chain represents myosin. Contraction occurs when calcium binds the troponin complex, allowing myosin to bind to actin with the production of force: "Myosin rows the actin sea". Reproduced with permission from Massachusetts Medical Society (Spirito P, Seidman CE, McKenna WJ et al. The management of hypertrophic cardiomyopathy. N Engl J Med 1997;336:775–85).

Protein	Percentage
Beta-myosin heavy chain	35
Myosin-binding protein C	15
Troponin T	15
Alpha-tropomyosin	1
Myosin light chain	1

Table 1. Mutations known to cause hypertrophic cardiomyopathy.

myocardial fiber disarray. Clearly, this cannot be a useful diagnostic marker during life, and increasing attention is being given to molecular genetic diagnostic tools.

Regardless of the electrocardiogram (ECG) presentation, the prognosis for HCM patients can be unpredictable. Some with severe hypertrophy remain asymptomatic, while others with apparently less severe hypertrophy develop arrhythmias, increased ventricular stiffness, heart failure, or sudden death. Indeed, there can be considerable variation in phenotype within families (see **Figure 2**).

Cardiomyopathy

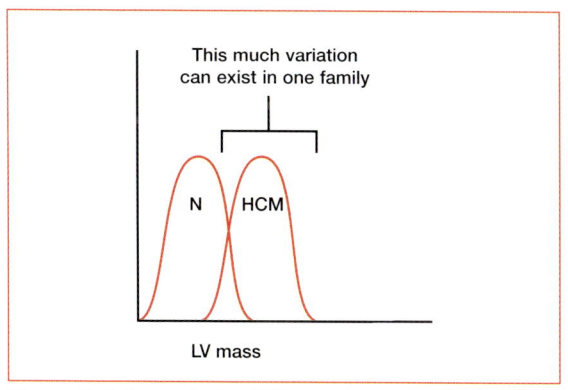

Figure 2. Left ventricular (LV) mass in a normal (N) individual and in a patient with hypertrophic cardiomyopathy (HCM).

Clinical examination
HCM has classic clinical signs, most of which relate to outflow obstruction (hence their presence is not required for diagnosis). They are as follows:

- jerky pulse
- prominent "a" wave in jugular venous pressure (JVP)
- double apex beat
- S3
- S4
- late ejection quality systolic murmur over the aortic area that is increased by standing and decreased by squatting
- a pansystolic murmur at the apex (indicating mitral regurgitation [MR])

The ECG may show LVH and T-wave inversion. With progressive left ventricular disease, left bundle branch block (LBBB) may appear.

Echo is the test of choice. Left ventricular wall thickness is measured from M-mode traces (see Chapter 4, Understanding the echocardiogram). Left ventricular outflow tract velocities can be measured and pressure drop estimated by continuous-wave Doppler. Diastolic dysfunction is common in HCM.

Specialist management
Medical
The main aim of medical treatment is to limit the effects of outflow tract obstruction. Beta-blockers and/or rate limiting calcium-channel blockers, such as verapamil, can improve diastolic filling (by reducing heart rate), reduce exercise-related outflow obstruction, and reduce the possibility of arrhythmia. Amiodarone

Chapter 11

and sotalol can prevent supraventricular and ventricular arrhythmia, but should only be used in patients with a previous episode.

Dual-chamber pacing
Patients who remain symptomatic despite drug therapy can have a DDD pacemaker inserted (see Chapter 8, Arrhythmia), set to a short atrioventricular (AV) delay. The effect of this is to pace the right ventricle each beat and induce an LBBB-type activation of the left ventricle, which reduces outflow obstruction by desynchronizing contraction of the septum and the posterior wall. Patients can be treadmill-tested to confirm that the AV delay is sufficiently short to maintain right ventricle capture at higher heart rates.

Nonsurgical septal reduction
A recent technique involving cardiac catheterization has been proposed as an alternative for outflow tract pressure gradient reduction and symptom improvement. This technique came to light following observations, in the early eighties, that upon balloon inflation in the left anterior descending (LAD) coronary artery there is a reduction of outflow tract velocities and gradients. The procedure involves balloon inflation in the proximal segment of the first septal perforator of the LAD and assessment of outflow tract gradient. If the gradient drops significantly, a small quantity of alcohol (3–5 mL) is injected down the cannulated artery, distal to the balloon, in an attempt to induce a localized proximal septal infarction. The velocities are then measured.

The stress-induced outflow tract gradient after dobutamine injection is also assessed, both before and after the procedure. If the results are not satisfactory, these steps are repeated while cannulating the second perforator of the LAD. Procedural success is always associated with significant myocardial enzyme rise and a fall in outflow tract velocities, development of significant conduction disturbance, and septal incoordinate relaxation. Mid- and long-term follow-up after nonsurgical septal reduction have proved promising in terms of a decrease in symptoms and maintained low outflow tract gradient.

Surgery
Until the last decade, the major nonmedical option for treating HCM with persistent symptoms was surgical myotomy/myectomy. In this procedure, which is also called the "Morrow procedure", a small portion of the proximal septal myocardium is resected to widen the outflow tract. Mortality from this technique is now <2% and there is a subjective symptomatic improvement in 70% of patients. However, complications are common and for the majority of patients it results in complete LBBB or they require a permanent pacemaker for complete heart block. As a consequence, surgeons have explored other possibilities, such as

History	Examination
Family history of premature death	Auscultate the heart, both lying and standing, with particular attention to outflow murmurs
Family history of heart disease at age <50 years	
Personal history of murmur, hypertension, excessive fatigability, or syncope	Assess radiofemoral delay to exclude coarctation
	Recognize the stigmata of Marfan's syndrome
Personal history of excessive or progressive shortness of breath or pain on exertion	Measure systemic blood pressure

Table 2. Key points in history and examination for preparticipation screening in athletes.

mitral valve replacement and anterior leaflet extension, to reduce MR, reduce outflow obstruction, and stiffen the anterior leaflet.

Preparticipation screening for sport

HCM is occasionally discovered during preparticipation screening for sport, and should be considered when a young athlete presents with voltage criteria LVH. In this situation, the question as to when to refer for echocardiography arises. The most common voltage criterion is that of Sokolow–Lyon (SV1 + RV5 >3.5 mV) (see Chapter 3, Conquering the ECG). Although the vast majority of young athletes in this category will have a normal heart, most cardiologists would recommend that any young, normotensive patient who meets these voltage criteria should be referred for an echo.

The ECG and echo are the key diagnostic tools. However, the overall prevalence of relevant conditions (0.2%) makes these cost-ineffective. Approximately 200 screenings are required to detect one abnormality, while 200,000 are needed to prevent one death. Thus, it is important to maximize the information available from history and examination (see **Table 2**).

There is consensus that history and physical examination are the only cost-effective screening tools for sudden cardiac death in athletes. However, these are very poor at identifying the primary causes of sudden death:

- HCM in its nonobstructive form (~35%) produces no murmur (see **Figure 3**)
- coronary artery abnormalities (~20%) are not detectable by simple clinical examination

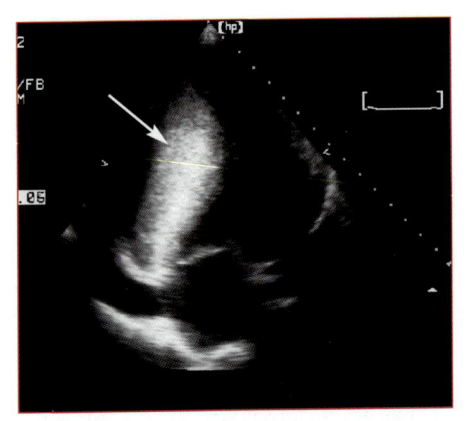

Figure 3. Hypertrophic nonobstructive cardiomyopathy. Note the grossly hypertrophied interventricular septum.

ECG patterns are distinctly abnormal (LVH, inverted T waves, deep Q waves, axis deviation, or LBBB) in about 15% of athletes, and mildly abnormal (borderline LVH, flat T wave, long PR interval, right bundle branch block) in another 25%. Early repolarization may account for another 15%. Bradycardia <60 bpm is found in more than a third. Abnormalities are most common in males younger than 20 years who are involved in endurance sports such as cycling, rowing, and cross-country skiing. In one series, 5% of over 1,000 consecutively examined athletes had structural abnormalities such as HCM or dilated cardiomyopathy (DCM).

Dilated cardiomyopathy

DCM is a primary disease of the cardiac muscle and can be defined as left or right ventricular dilatation and failure in the absence of coronary artery disease, hypertension, valve disease, or congenital heart abnormality. Patients usually present with shortness of breath and signs of congestion in an identical way to heart failure of any other cause. There are many causes of DCM:

- alcohol
- familial
- myocarditis
- postradiation or chemotherapy (eg, adriamycin/doxorubicin)
- hemochromatosis
- thyrotoxicosis
- thiamine deficiency

Prognosis
The prognosis is variable according to the degree of ventricular damage. It is generally agreed that patients with resistant high filling pressures do badly. Those with biventricular dilatation and impairment of function do even worse.

Investigations
The ECG shows no specific signs: it may be normal or show conduction disturbances. Chest x-ray shows increased cardiothoracic ratio and pulmonary vascular congestion.

Echo is the test of choice and will show a grossly dilated ventricle with thin walls and globally impaired systolic function. Disease progression results in functional MR and the development of left atrial dilatation. In rare cases, the disease solely affects the right heart. Cardiac catheterization is used to exclude coronary artery disease and measure intracardiac pressures.

Management
Management is as described for chronic heart failure (see Chapter 7, Heart failure).

Restrictive cardiomyopathy

Restrictive cardiomyopathy is a disease of the heart muscle that results in myocardial stiffness and an incompliant ventricle. Patients present with predominantly right-sided failure (gross peripheral edema, raised JVP, hepatomegaly) and a normal-sized heart. Classic clinical signs are rapid x and y descent of the JVP, and loud S3 and S4.

The most common causes are:

- hemochromatosis
- sarcoidosis
- amyloidosis
- carcinoid syndrome
- glycogen storage disease
- scleroderma
- endomyocardial fibrosis and eosinophilic heart disease

Investigations
The ECG can be a useful tool, as subendocardial fibrosis can result in conduction disturbances. In addition, amyloid heart disease presents with low voltages. However, echo enables diagnosis. Classic findings include:

- absence of ventricular dilatation or hypertrophy (common but not invariable)
- left ventricle and right ventricle systolic function are often normal
- there may be biatrial dilatation
- the myocardium may be speckled or echogenic
- the Doppler ventricular in-flow pattern exhibits a high E:A ratio (see Chapter 4, Understanding the echocardiogram)

The key differential diagnosis is constrictive pericarditis. This is an important distinction to make as constrictive pericarditis can be treated surgically.

Management

There is no specific medical treatment for restrictive cardiomyopathy. The main aim is to control symptoms of cardiac failure. In patients with high filling pressures, angiotensin-converting enzyme inhibitors in particular have shown a significant beneficial effect in unloading the left ventricle and improving symptoms. Atrial fibrillation should be controlled with digoxin and a prophylactic anticoagulant is usually recommended.

Eosinophilic cardiomyopathy can be treated with steroids, cytotoxic drugs, and prophylactic anticoagulants for thromboembolism. Endomyocardial fibrosis that is not controlled by medical therapy may warrant surgical intervention for subendocardial decortication. Carcinoid syndrome may require tricuspid valve replacement (see Chapter 9, Valve disease).

Further reading

Maron BJ, Moller JH, Seidman C et al. Impact of laboratory molecular diagnosis on contemporary diagnostic criteria for genetically transmitted cardiovascular disease: hypertrophic cardiomyopathy, long-QT syndrome, and Marfan Syndrome. *Circulation* 1998;98:1460–71.

Pelliccia A, Maron BJ, Culasso F et al. Clinical significance of abnormal electrocardiographic patterns in trained athletes. *Circulation* 2000;102:278–84.

Prior SG, Aliot E, Blomstrom-Lundqvist C et al. Task force on sudden cardiac death of the European Society of Cardiology. *Eur Heart J* 2001;22:1374–450.

Chapter 12

Aneurysm and dissection of the aorta

Aortic aneurysm

Aneurysms of the thoracic aorta (see **Figure 1**) are not as common as those affecting the abdominal portion, but carry a higher risk of rupture. Both share the same primary cause: atherosclerosis. In the past, ascending aortic aneurysms were typically caused by syphilis, but nowadays hypertension or Marfan's syndrome are more likely to be responsible. Symptoms result from the acute painful tear felt as central chest pain, which radiates to the back, and from the compression of surrounding structures:

- dysphagia (esophagus)
- dyspnea (bronchi; pericardial effusion)
- upper thorax/neck swelling (superior vena cava)

Standard radiology and echocardiography can be useful in monitoring the progression of aneurysms. Computed tomography (CT) is the gold standard and should be carried out annually in patients with known disease that does not yet require surgery or percutaneous placement of an aortic prosthesis/stents. However, magnetic resonance imaging (MRI) is increasingly being used.

Management
The central feature of management is rigorous control of blood pressure (BP). Therapy should include a β-blocker and be aimed at keeping systolic pressure <120 mm Hg.

Marfan's syndrome
Described by Bernard Marfan in 1896, this autosomal dominant single-gene disorder results from a mutation of the fibrillin gene on chromosome 15. The key clinical features are:

- arachnodactyly (long spindly fingers)
- high-arched palate
- pectus excavatum

Chapter 12

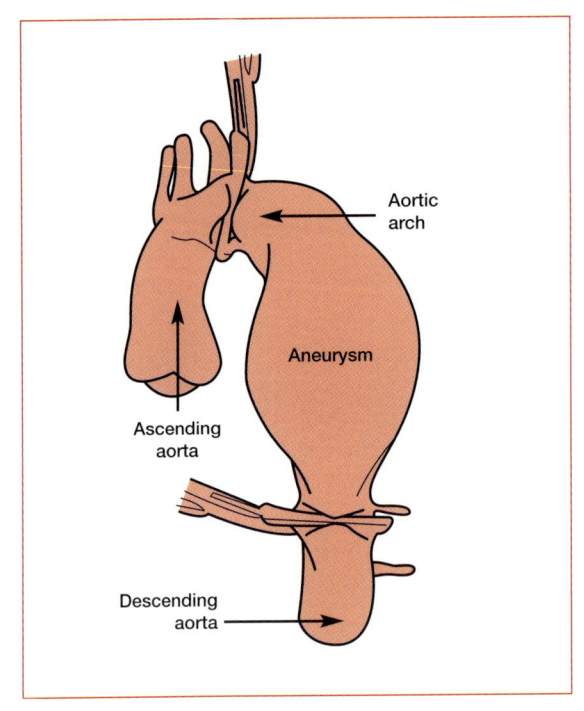

Figure 1. A typical aneurysm of the thoracic aorta at surgery.

ABRAHAM LINCOLN

Abraham Lincoln was both tall (6 ft 4 in) and thin (160–180 lb). He had long arms and legs, and large, narrow hands and feet. Contemporary descriptions of his appearance indicate that he was stoop-shouldered, loose-jointed, and walked with a shuffling gait. In addition, he wore eyeglasses to correct a visual problem. It is not surprising then that many have concluded that he suffered from Marfan's syndrome. Certainly, he shared a great-great-grandfather with a man who had a confirmed diagnosis of Marfan's. In fact, this observation, reported by Dr Harold Schwartz in 1959, was the beginning of a mystery that has taxed historians and doctors ever since. However, Lincoln showed few other signs of Marfan's. He had visual problems, but examination of his eyeglasses reveals he was farsighted and not nearsighted – a classic symptom of Marfan's. Also, a cast of his hands has shown that they were muscular and powerful, and not the slender hands of someone with Marfan's syndrome. Although the fun of the mystery is often in the debate and not in the answer, this is one theory that could be tested: a limited amount of bone fragments and hair from Lincoln was retained by the attending physician at the time of his assassination. Molecular testing using these samples could end the debate in an instant.

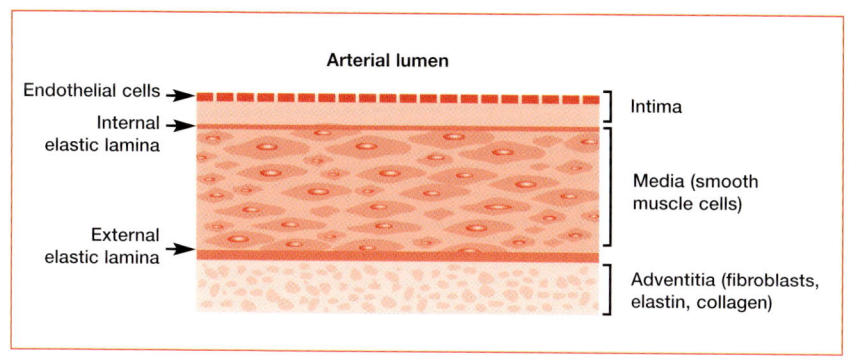

Figure 2. The adventitia, media, and intima of the aortic wall.

- an armspan greater than height
- upward lens dislocation
- aortic root dilatation and aortic incompetence
- mitral valve prolapse

The key differential diagnosis is homocystinuria, a recessively inherited defect in amino-acid metabolism, which has similar skeletal features. Homocystinuria is associated with low IQ and typically causes downward dislocation of the lens. However, it does not affect the heart.

Marfan's patients should undergo annual echo screening of the aortic root and prophylactic replacement should be considered when the diameter reaches 55 mm (a normal diameter is 40 mm). Beta-blockade can retard the rate of dilatation, but patients who do not have the replacement die in the fourth or fifth decade from aortic dissection or cardiac failure secondary to aortic regurgitation.

Sinus of Valsalva
A congenital aneurysm of the sinus of Valsalva is a rare cause of arteriovenous shunt. It is formed because of a weak connection between the aortic valve and the aortic fibrous ring. This enlarges during childhood and usually ruptures in adulthood into the right ventricle, creating a volume shunt from the left to the right side of the heart. The diagnosis is confirmed by aortography. Without surgical repair, biventricular failure results.

Aortic dissection

Dissection, which is usually caused by atherosclerosis, is the development of a tear in the aortic intima that creates a false lumen through the aortic media for a variable distance (see **Figures 2** and **3**).

Chapter 12

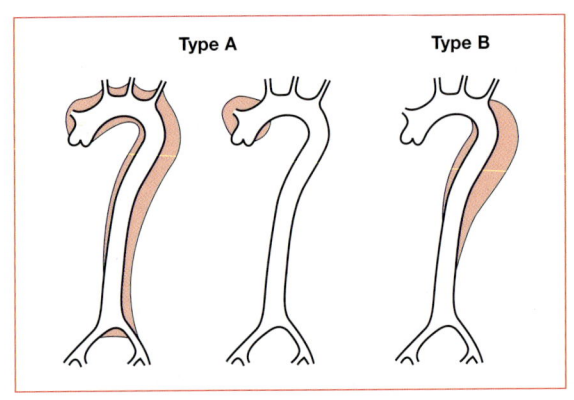

Figure 3. Classification of dissection.

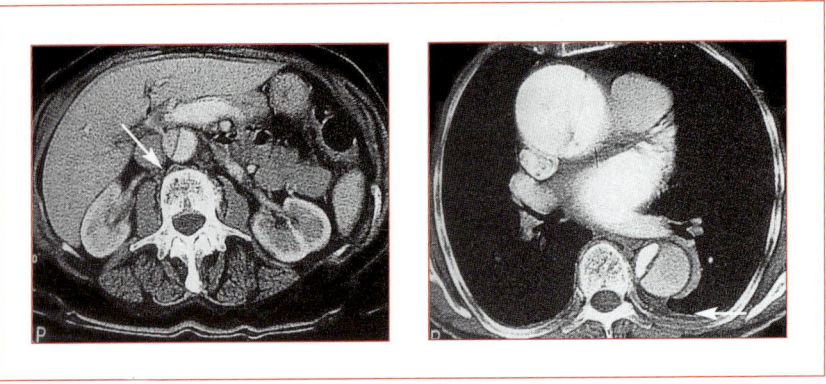

Figure 4. Computed tomography scans showing dissection of the aorta.

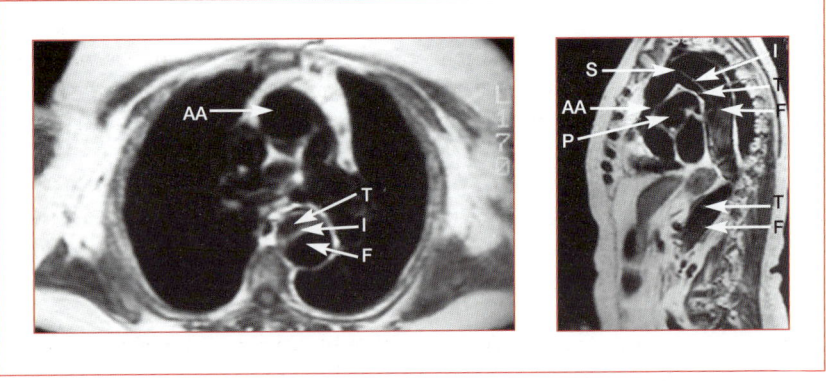

Figure 5. Magnetic resonance images showing separation of the dissected membrane. AA: ascending aorta; F: false lumen; I: intimal flap; P: pulmonary artery; S: subclavian artery; T: true lumen.

Aneurysm and dissection of the aorta

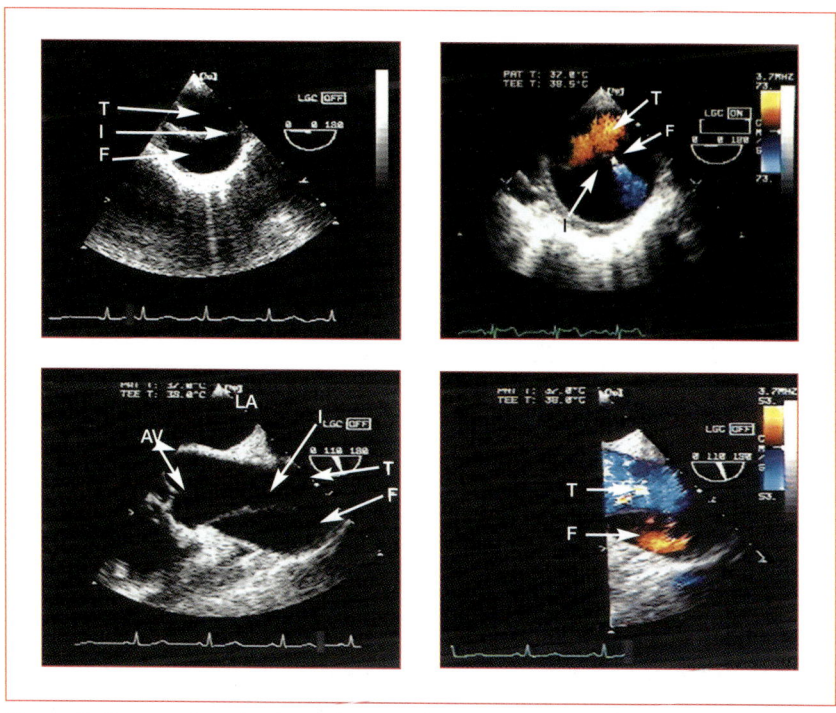

Figure 6. Transesophageal echocardiograms showing separation of the dissecting membrane. AV: aortic valve; F: false lumen; I: intimal flap; LA: left atrium; T: true lumen.

Dissection is classified according to whether it includes the ascending aorta (type A) or not (type B) (see **Figure 3**). Type A dissection is a surgical emergency because of the high risk of proximal extension, rupture, and sudden death. If a type A dissection is confirmed by CT or MRI, the patient should be operated on immediately. The highly specialized repair operation can involve replacement of the aortic root with a vascular graft, reimplantation of the coronary arteries, and resuspension of the aortic valve. In some cases it may be necesssary to replace the valve.

In contrast, type B dissection is managed medically by aggressive antihypertensive treatment. In the acute situation, the systolic BP should be lowered to <110 mm Hg using intravenous (IV) β-blockade (eg, labetalol). Beta-blockade, as well as reducing the BP, reduces the BP's rate of rise and for this reason it is preferred to sodium nitroprusside as the first-line IV agent. If β-blockers are contraindicated then rate-limiting calcium-channel blockers, such as diltiazem or verapamil, can be used.

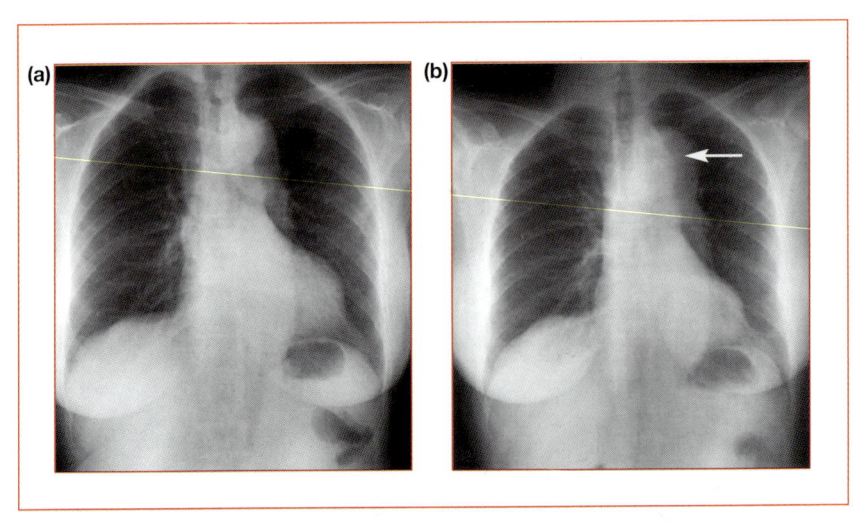

Figure 7. (**a**,**b**) Chest x-rays. A dissected aorta can be seen in (**b**) (arrow).

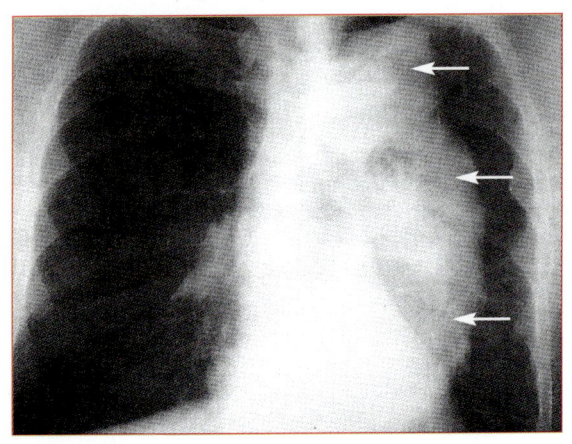

Figure 8. Chest x-ray showing extreme dissection of the aorta (arrows).

Dissection typically presents with a severe tearing central chest pain that radiates to the back. A patient with such a history should be referred urgently to a specialist center since the ascending aorta might be involved. Immediate investigations include:

- CT or MRI scan (see **Figures 4** and **5**, previous page)
- transesophageal echo to assess possible aortic regurgitation (see **Figure 6**, previous page)
- transthoracic echo for pericardial effusion
- preoperatively, coronary artery disease must be ruled out by coronary angiography

A physical examination can prove useful diagnostically, but should not delay the above emergency investigations. It should include:

- measurement of the BP in both arms (unequal BP is a sign, though not a reliable sign)
- documentation of all peripheral pulses (lack of peripheral pulses may be the only sign if the dissection spares the ascending aorta)
- close attention to heart sounds (aortic regurgitation and tamponade are possible with proximal extension)
- neurologic examination (hemiplegia or paraplegia can result from occlusion of the carotid arteries and anterior spinal arteries, respectively)

Other potentially useful investigations are:

- assessment of renal function, including urine microscopy and catheterization for accurate measurement of renal output
- a chest x-ray, which often shows a distended aorta or generalized widening of the mediastinum (see **Figures 7** and **8**)

Further reading

Erbel R, Alfonso F, Boileau C et al.; Task Force on Aortic Dissection, European Society of Cardiology. Diagnosis and management of aortic dissection. *Eur Heart J* 2001;22:1642–81.

Khan IA, Nair CK. Clinical, diagnostic, and management perspectives of aortic dissection. *Chest* 2002;122:311–28.

Chapter 13

Pericardial disease

Pericarditis

A diagnosis of pericarditis (inflammation of the pericardium), though rare, should always be considered as a differential for ischemic heart pain. The key differentiating features are that the pain in pericarditis is altered by posture and can be exacerbated by deep inspiration. Classically, the patient will be found sitting forward and taking shallow breaths.

Pathophysiology

The pericardium has two layers: visceral and parietal. The visceral layer is closely apposed to the heart, whilst the fibrous parietal layer provides a more rigid outer shell to the pericardial cavity (see **Figure 1**). The normal volume of pericardial fluid is in the region of 50 mL.

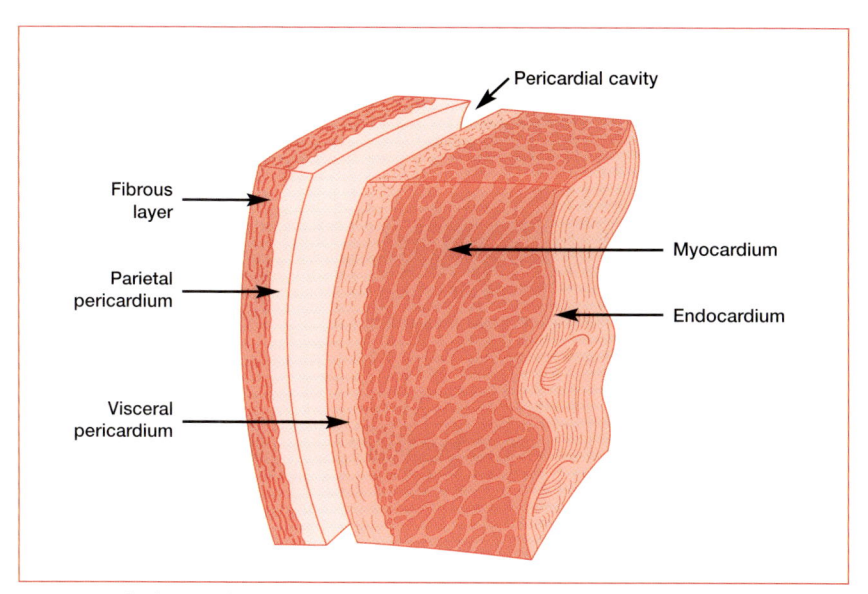

Figure 1. The layers of pericardium. The visceral pericardium is a tissue paper-like layer, while the parietal pericardium is more rigid.

Chapter 13

Causes of pericarditis
Postmyocardial infarction/postcardiac surgery
Viral (Coxsackie B, influenza)
Metastatic malignancy
Uremia
Tuberculous
Systemic lupus erythematosus

Table 1. Causes of pericarditis.

The causes of pericarditis are outlined in **Table 1**. Viral pericarditis is the most common type, but in many cases either the diagnosis is never made or the viral infection is never identified. Another common presentation is characteristic pain 3–14 days postmyocardial infarction (MI) or postcardiac surgery, which tends to be self-limiting. Relapsing episodes are referred to as Dressler's syndrome or postcardiotomy syndrome, and are thought to represent an autoimmune process.

Investigations
Examination
Auscultation may reveal a pericardial rub, which is sufficient, but not necessary, to make the diagnosis. It can easily be distinguished from a pleural rub by asking the patient to hold their breath.

Electrocardiography
The classic sign of pericarditis – a concave upwards ("saddle") ST-segment elevation throughout the 12 leads – is, of course, rare. However, some form of electrocardiogram (ECG) abnormality is common. These changes are either present in all 12 leads or in leads that do not correspond to the territory perfused by a single coronary artery. Low voltages suggest the possibility of effusion.

Chest x-ray
A chest x-ray (CXR) can help to rule out a tuberculous cause of pericarditis and exclude significant effusion.

Echocardiography
Echocardiography is helpful mainly if there is a suspicion of effusion or tamponade.

Blood tests
Blood tests for immune markers, such as the antinuclear cytoplasmic antibody (ANCA), should be carried out in any patient with confirmed pericarditis. Acute and convalescent viral titers can also be requested, but rarely alter management.

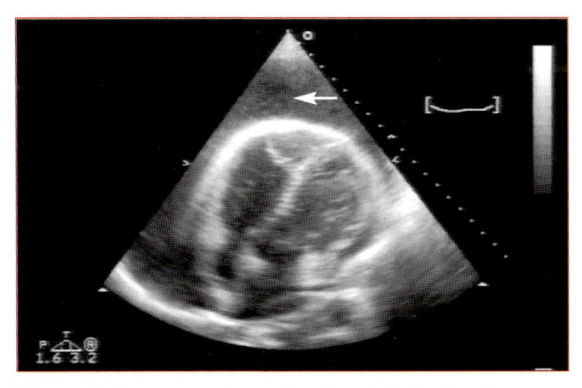

Figure 2. An extreme form of pericardial effusion, known as a "swinging heart". The arrow indicates the effusion.

Management
Nonsteroidal anti-inflammatory drugs are the treatment of choice for pericarditis. They relieve both the inflammatory process and the pain. Steroids may be required in serositic pericarditis, whereas pericarditis with a suspicious CXR and constitutional symptoms should prompt investigation for tuberculosis.

Pericardial effusion and tamponade

As with pleural effusion, the key defining presentation of pericardial effusion is the rate of fluid accumulation. Any cause of pericarditis can result in a significant accumulation of serous fluid, while hemopericardium (a collection of blood in the pericardial sac surrounding the heart) can be caused by trauma, type 1 dissection of the aorta, and cardiac rupture. The key feature is not the overall volume of fluid (even hundreds of milliliters can be asymptomatic if accumulated over a long enough time), but the rate of rise – as with pleural effusion, removal of even a small amount of fluid can result in significant benefit.

Small, asymptomatic effusions can often be left to resorb on their own. This usually requires repeat echo at regular intervals to ensure that resorption has occurred. Larger effusions bounded by the tough parietal pericardium can compromise the low pressure right heart – this results in tamponade (see **Figure 2**).

Examination
Cardiac tamponade is a medical emergency. It is associated with a characteristic jugular venous pressure (JVP). Kussmaul's sign describes a raised JVP that rises further on inspiration, while Friedrich's sign describes a steep x/y descent (although, in reality at the bedside, the waves are hard to discern). The heart sounds are quiet and there may be a rub.

> **KUSSMAUL'S LEGACY**
> *Adolph Kussmaul was Professor of Medicine successively at Heidelberg, Erlangen, Freiburg, and Strasbourg. As well as describing the paradoxical increase in JVP on inspiration in patients with restrictive cardiomyopathy, right ventricular failure, and constrictive pericarditis, he described the deep-sighing respiration associated with low arterial pH (Kussmaul breathing) and coined the term "polyarteritis nodosa". In fact, Kussmaul's JVP sign is widely misunderstood to be solely the result of right ventricular incompliance, when in fact the explanation relates as much to distension of the mesenteric vascular bed and the change from a right ventricular pressure that predominantly reflects negative intrapleural pressure "sucking" blood into the chest, to one that predominantly reflects positive intra-abdominal pressure "pushing" the greater volume proximally.*

A characteristic of cardiac tamponade is pulsus paradoxus, which is not paradoxical at all, but an exaggeration of the normal drop in systolic pressure on inspiration – >10 mm Hg is abnormal. To test for it, inflate the cuff to just above systolic pressure then slowly deflate, stopping each 5 mm Hg for a full inspiration–expiration cycle. Listen for the point at which the beating becomes continuous throughout the breathing cycle.

Electrocardiography
Low-voltage ECG and beat-to-beat variation in R-wave amplitude are characteristic.

Chest x-ray
CXRs show a globular, "boot-shaped" heart.

Echocardiography
Echo is the investigation of choice. The key observation is diastolic collapse of the right atrium and ventricle. It demands urgent pericardiocentesis.

Constrictive pericarditis

In constrictive pericarditis, the pericardium becomes rigid and fibrotic, adheres to the myocardium, and limits its function. It most commonly follows tuberculous pericarditis or hemopericardium, but can result from any cause of pericarditis.

The classic clinical picture is:

- significant ascites
- raised JVP with positive Kussmaul and Friedrich's signs
- hepatomegaly
- pulsus paradoxus (but usually less severe than in tamponade)
- pericardial knock (high-pitched early diastolic added sound)
- calcification visible on the lateral CXR

The most difficult differential diagnosis is restrictive cardiomyopathy. However, the left ventricular function is usually preserved in constrictive pericarditis, and filling pressures are raised. The only treatment for constrictive pericarditis is surgical excision of the pericardium.

Chapter 14

Adult congenital heart disease

Congenital abnormalities of the heart and cardiovascular system are reported in almost 1% of live births (see **Figure 1**) and about half of these children need medical or surgical help during infancy. In the first decade, a further 25% require surgery to maintain or improve their life. Only 10% survive to adolescence without surgery. Of these 10%, however, many live a normal life for years before their abnormality is discovered.

Recognizing adult congenital heart disease

There are a few signs that should alert generalists to the possibility of congenital heart disease:

- murmurs, especially continuous – there are few degenerative diseases that produce continuous murmurs
- cyanosis, clubbing – unless there is coexistent lung disease, a patient with a murmur and cyanosis should be referred for echocardiography
- right bundle branch block (RBBB) – this occurs in 1% of the middle-aged population without disease. When combined with a murmur, the patient should be referred for echocardiography

In most cases, suspicion of congenital heart disease leads to a cardiology referral. However, an awareness of the possible diagnoses will help your referral.

Ventricular septal defect

Ventricular septal defect (VSD) (see **Figures 2** and **3**) is the most common congenital heart defect. Symptoms depend on the size of the defect and the age of the patient. Small VSDs are usually asymptomatic and compatible with a normal life (in fact, about 40% close spontaneously in early childhood). Large VSDs cause cardiac failure in the second or third month after birth. If a large shunt does not produce symptoms during infancy, there is usually little disturbance until late adolescence or early adult life when the patient develops high pulmonary vascular resistance, breathlessness, fatigue, and cyanosis. There is progression to effort syncope, recurrent hemoptysis, and heart failure.

Chapter 14

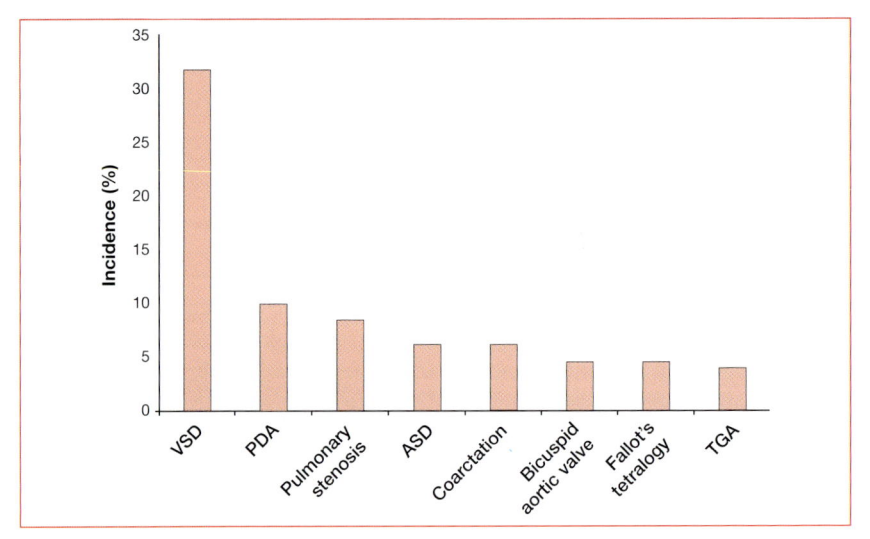

Figure 1. The relative incidence of common congenital heart defects. ASD: atrial septal defect; PDA: patent ductus arteriosus; TGA: transposition of the great arteries; VSD: ventricular septal defect.

Recognizing VSD

In VSD patients, the apex beat may be hyperdynamic and there could be a systolic thrill. The classic sign is a loud pansystolic murmur, often accompanied by a mid diastolic murmur at the apex (due to high flow through the mitral valve) (see Table 1). In patients with raised pulmonary vascular resistance, right ventricular hypertrophy (RVH) is evident and the pulmonary second sound might be accentuated, followed by the early diastolic murmur of pulmonary regurgitation.

With small VSDs, the electrocardiogram (ECG) is normal. With larger ones, there is evidence of biventricular enlargement (tall R waves and deep S waves in leads V1–V6), especially when pulmonary vascular resistance is high. Similarly, with a small defect the chest x-ray (CXR) is normal, but with a large shunt there is cardiomegaly and prominence of the pulmonary vessels.

Large shunts should be closed surgically. However, if pulmonary hypertension has developed, surgery is usually contraindicated as closing it may worsen the pulmonary hypertension.

The main complication of VSD is infective endocarditis. Vegetations may appear at the tricuspid valve, opposite or around the defect, or on the aortic valve. In certain lesions, aortic incompetence may develop due to loss of support of the valve.

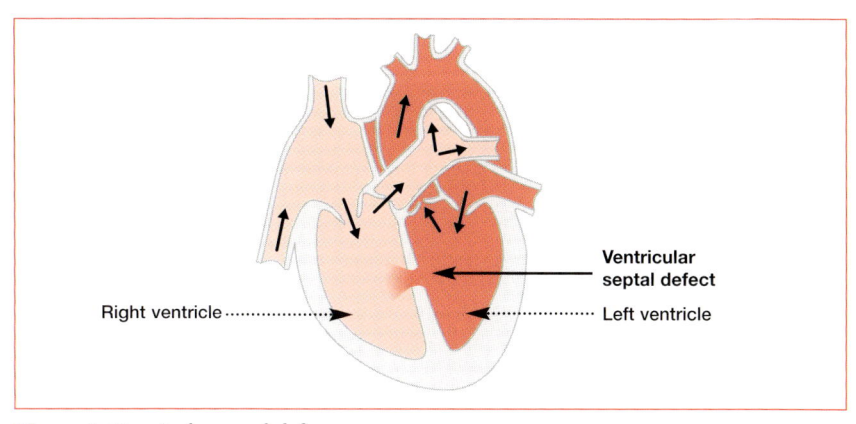

Figure 2. Ventricular septal defect.

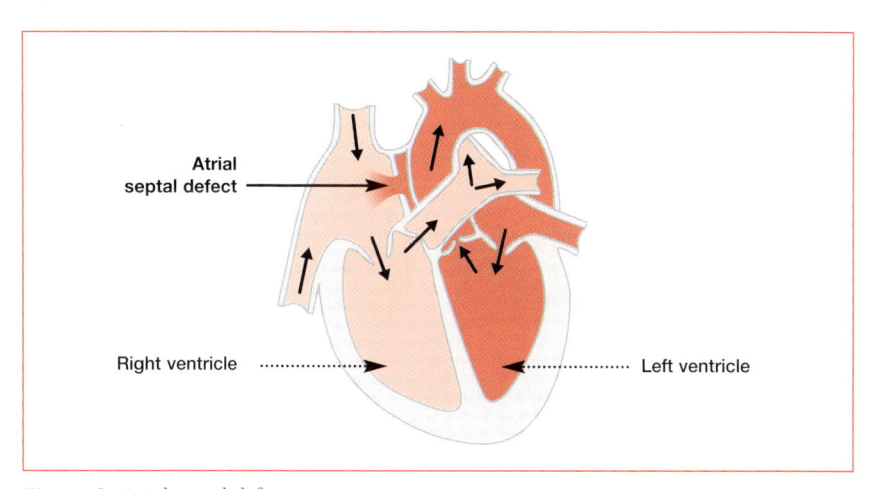

Figure 3. Atrial septal defect.

The prognosis for adults with uncomplicated VSD is good. Few patients have defects large enough to cause serious hemodynamic problems, but all are exposed to the risk of infective endocarditis.

Atrial septal defect

Three types of atrial septal defect (ASD) can occur:

- ostium secundum is the most common type (70%). It can be large, but usually does not affect the atrioventricular valves (see **Figures 3** and **4**)
- ostium primum – the hole is situated close to the atrioventricular valves and can be associated with an atrioventricular septal defect

Ventricular septal defect	Atrial septal defect
Biventricular hypertrophy RVH	LAD, RBBB (primum) RVH, RAD, RBBB (secundum)
PSM	MSM (MDM)

Table 1. Characteristics of atrial septal defect and ventricular septal defect. Note the wide, fixed splitting of the second heart sound in atrial septal defect. LAD: left axis deviation; MDM: mid diastolic murmur; MSM: mid systolic murmur; PSM: pansystolic accentuation of murmur; RAD: right axis deviation; RBBB: right bundle branch block; RVH: right ventricular hypertrophy.

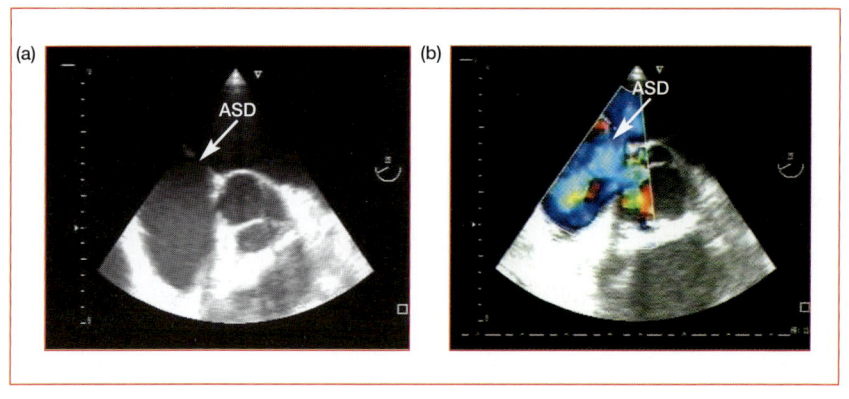

Figure 4. Atrial septal defect (ASD) shown by (**a**) transesophageal echocardiography, and (**b**) transesophageal Doppler.

- sinus venosus is a defect situated near the entrance of the superior vena cava (SVC) or inferior vena cava to the right atrium. It is unusual and is often associated with partial anomalous pulmonary venous drainage (usually drainage of the right upper lobe into the SVC)

Pathophysiology
The shunt of blood from the left atrium to the right atrium results in:

- increased volume load and dilatation of the right atrium and right ventricle (RV)
- increased pulmonary blood flow and enlargement of the pulmonary arteries
- increase in size of the pulmonary veins
- reduced filling of the left ventricle (LV) and aorta

Over time, the aorta and LV shrink, and pulmonary vascular resistance increases and causes Eisenmenger syndrome (see below).

Recognizing ASD

Most patients with secundum ASD remain asymptomatic throughout their thirties, but visit their doctor in middle-age with the onset of breathlessness and fatigue (note the nonspecific signs). Symptoms are usually progressive and worsened by the development of atrial arrhythmias. Patients with primum ASD tend to present earlier and with more severe symptoms.

The classic sign of ASD is wide, fixed splitting of the second heart sound, together with a systolic murmur due to high flow across the pulmonary valve (see **Table 1**). Primum ASD may be accompanied by mitral regurgitation.

ECG might indicate RBBB and either RVH and right axis deviation (secundum) or left axis deviation (primum) (see **Table 1**). CXR may show cardiomegaly with a prominent pulmonary trunk.

Management

ASDs that are large enough to give clear physical signs should be closed. Closure of an ostium secundum defect is relatively easy and carries a low mortality rate. Correction of an ostium primum defect, with its associated anomalies, is more difficult and carries a higher mortality rate. More recently, percutaneous device closure of small and moderate size ASDs has been possible. In this procedure, a "butterfly" device (eg, the Clamshell occluder, the Starflex occluder, or the Amplatzer occluder) is manipulated noninvasively into the heart and "opened", whereupon it grasps the defect on either side and closes it (see **Figures 5** and **6**).

Primum ASD requires prophylaxis for infective endocarditis, while secundum ASD does not.

Eisenmenger syndrome

This is the name given to reversal in the direction of a cardiac shunt caused by the development of pulmonary hypertension. It applies regardless of whether the shunt is atrial or ventricular. Initial flow is always from high pressure (left) to low pressure (right), but pulmonary pressure can rise above systemic pressure and cause a reversal of flow.

Signs of pulmonary hypertension are RVH, pulmonary systolic click, and loud pulmonary valve closure. CXR shows large main pulmonary arteries and branches with peripheral pruning. After the development of Eisenmenger physiology, only heart–lung transplantation is of value in management.

Chapter 14

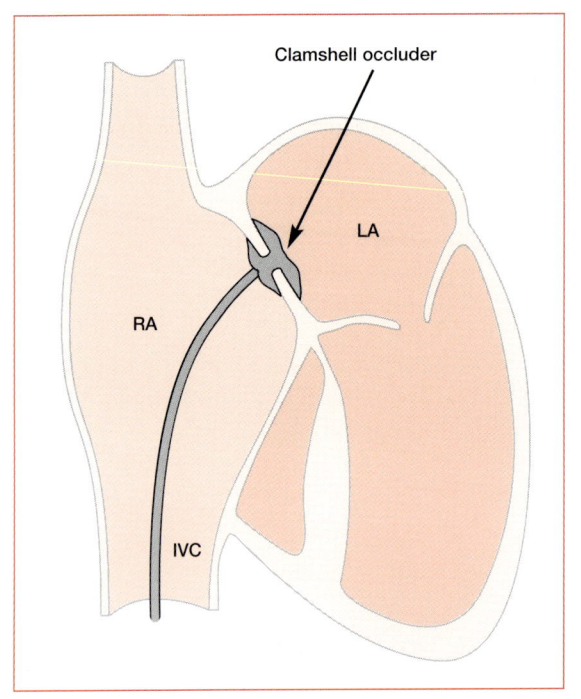

Figure 5. The Clamshell occluder for closure of an atrial septal defect. IVC: inferior vena cava; LA: left atrium; RA: right atrium.

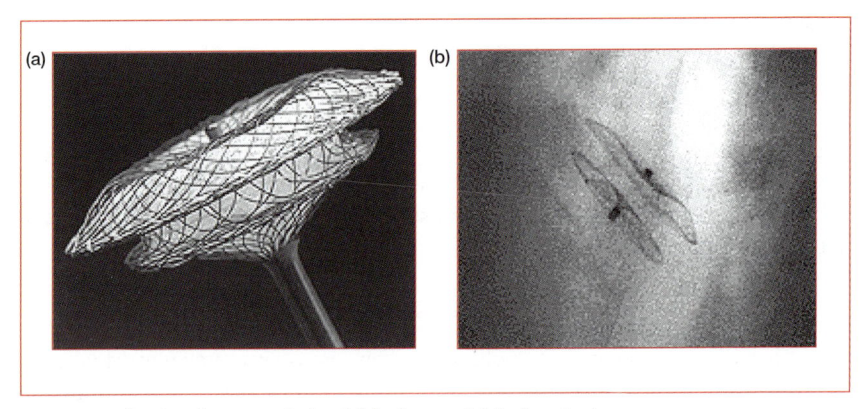

Figure 6. The Amplatzer occluder (**a**) before and (**b**) after deployment.

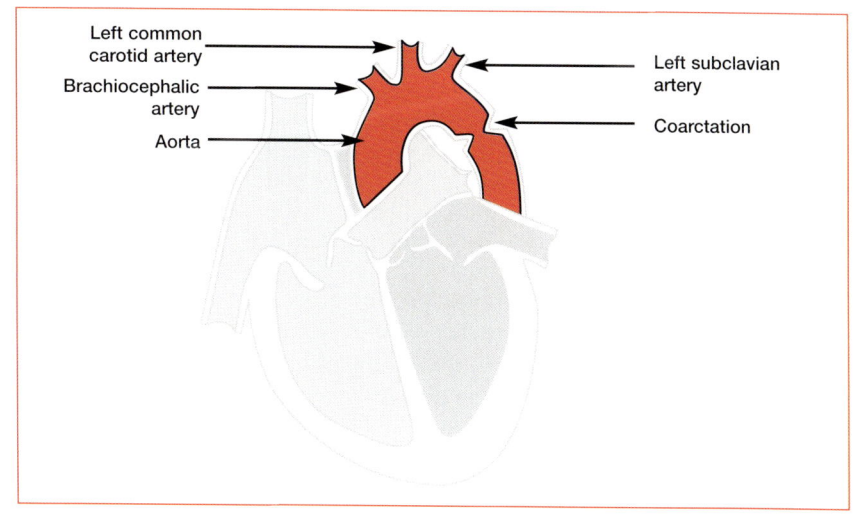

Figure 7. Coarctation of the aorta.

Bicuspid aortic valve

Bicuspid aortic valves often function normally throughout most of a patient's life. However, fibrosis and calcification ultimately lead to aortic stenosis (see Chapter 9, Valve disease) and an eventual requirement for surgical correction.

Coarctation of the aorta

Coarctation of the aorta is a narrowing of the lumen, usually just distal to the origin of the left subclavian artery (see **Figure 7**). Most commonly, the patient presents in their twenties or thirties, usually with hypertension. Without surgery, 50% die before the age of 30 years. Potential treatments include resection of the narrowed segment with end-to-end anastomosis, repair involving the subclavian artery, and balloon angioplasty – the role of which remains controversial. Hypertension, which is often the presenting feature, must be aggressively treated both before and after surgery (it commonly persists).

Pulmonary valve stenosis

Patients with mild to moderate pulmonary stenosis usually remain asymptomatic until the onset of atrial flutter/fibrillation or right heart failure, which lead to breathlessness, ascites, peripheral edema, and a visit to the doctor. Fatigue, slight dyspnea, and effort syncope occur with severe narrowing. The physical signs depend on the severity of the obstruction and secondary effects on RV function. In severe stenosis, the arterial pulse is small and the jugular venous pulse exhibits a large "a" wave. On palpation, there is nearly always a systolic thrill in the second left intercostal space and there is a left parasternal heave. An early systolic "ejection" click and a loud ejection murmur are best heard in the second intercostal space. The second sound is normal in mild cases, but in more severe cases it is widely split and the second (pulmonary) element is soft. ECG shows RVH in severe stenosis, while CXR shows a dilated pulmonary trunk with oligemic lung fields. Balloon valvotomy is indicated in severe pulmonary stenosis. Surgical valvotomy is an alternative.

Patent ductus arteriosus

Patent ductus arteriosus (PDA) describes a preservation of the connection between the pulmonary artery and the aorta that exists in the fetus (see **Figure 8**). Since aortic diastolic pressure is higher than pulmonary artery systolic pressure, there is continuous flow into the pulmonary circulation, creating the characteristic continuous ("machinery") murmur, heard best just below the left clavicle. In hemodynamically insignificant lesions (>50% of cases), patients are asymptomatic. Patients with bigger shunts develop cardiac failure at an age that depends on the severity of the lesion. Eisenmenger syndrome can occur with PDA. Treatment is surgical closure of the duct; this can be carried out percutaneously.

Fallot's tetralogy

Fallot's tetralogy is one of the causes of cyanotic congenital heart disease. The features derive from an abnormally positioned aorta that "over-rides" the interventricular septum (see **Figure 9**). This causes:

- perimembranous VSD
- RV outflow obstruction (pulmonary stenosis)
- RVH

The chief symptom is cyanosis on exercise. Children typically "squat" for relief of dyspnea after exercise (almost pathognomonic). Chest pain, arrhythmia, and congestive heart failure are more common in adults than in children. Clubbing is common. Surgical correction usually involves resection of the hypertrophied RV infundibulum and VSD closure with incorporation of the aorta into the RV. Adult Fallot's patients often suffer impaired exercise capacity due to poor RV function.

Transposition of the great arteries

In transposition of the great arteries (TGA), the RV connects to the aorta and the LV connects to the pulmonary artery (see **Figure 10**). The result, following peripartum closure of the foramen ovale, is two parallel circulations – a physiology that is not compatible with life. The neonate would die instantly were it not for the common coexistence of a patent foramen ovale, ASD, VSD, or PDA. In infants, an

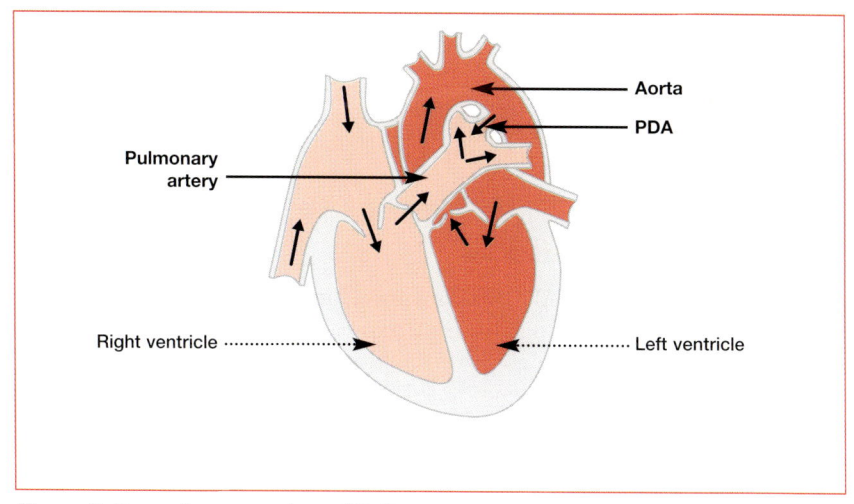

Figure 8. Patent ductus arteriosus (PDA).

improvement in symptoms can be achieved by creating a large defect in the atrial septum to allow mixing of the blood between systemic and pulmonary circulations (Rashkind's procedure – see **Figure 11**). This is performed by passing a balloon catheter into the left atrium via the right atrium. After inflation, the balloon catheter is pulled back forcefully into the right atrium, creating a tear in the septum. This procedure is usually effective in the neonatal period and allows the child to live until the latter part of the first year of life, when the Mustard operation can be performed. This involves rerouting venous return by inserting an intra-atrial baffle. The definitive treatment is the arterial switch operation, in which the arteries are switched back to their appropriate ventricles. The biggest challenge with this procedure is reattaching the coronary arteries, the anatomical organization of which is variable in TGA. In addition, the "low pressure" LV must take on filling of the systemic circulation.

Ebstein's anomaly

Ebstein's anomaly is the downward displacement of a portion of the tricuspid valve with atrialization of a large part of the RV (see **Figure 12**). There is often an associated ostium secundum ASD. The atrialized portion of the ventricle hinders rather than helps the forward flow of blood and there is tricuspid regurgitation. Occasionally Ebstein's anomaly is asymptomatic, but it generally presents in childhood or early adulthood with dyspnea, fatigue, signs of tricuspid regurgitation, and right-sided cardiac failure. Patients with Ebstein's anomaly require prophylaxis for endocarditis.

Chapter 14

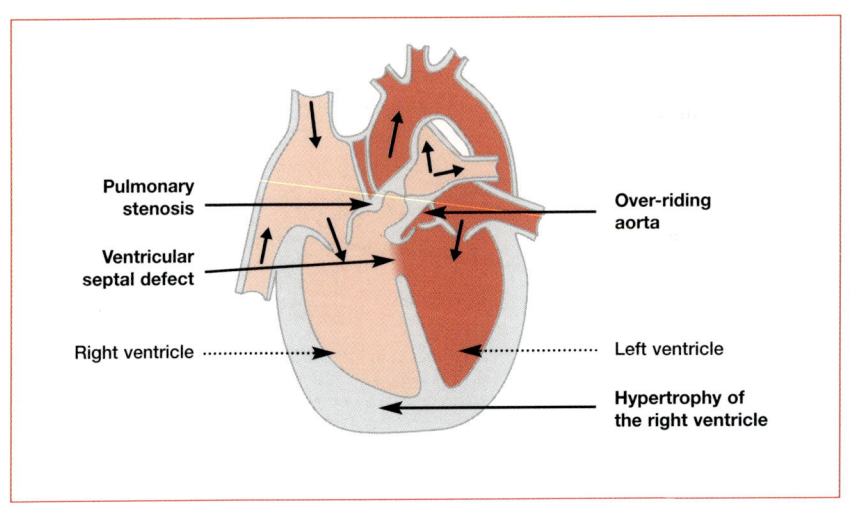

Figure 9. Fallot's tetralogy with an "over-riding aorta".

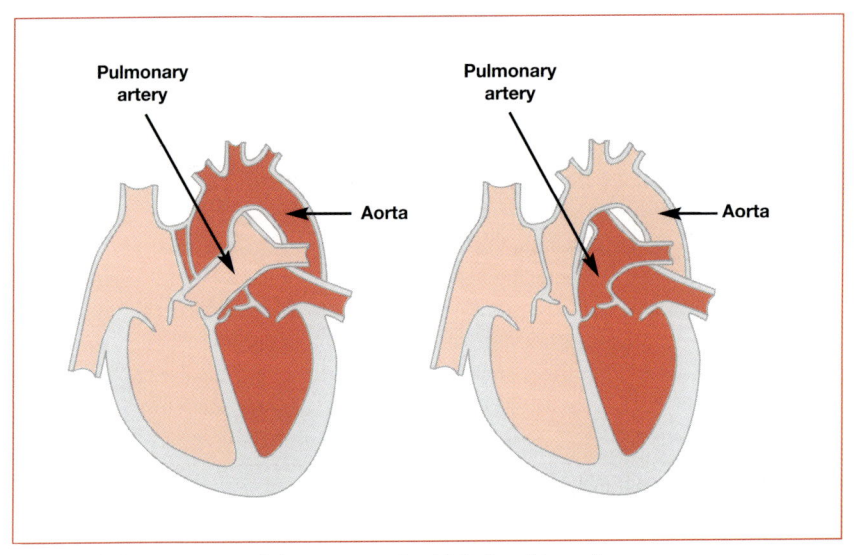

Figure 10. Transposition of the great arteries (right-hand image).

212

Adult congenital heart disease

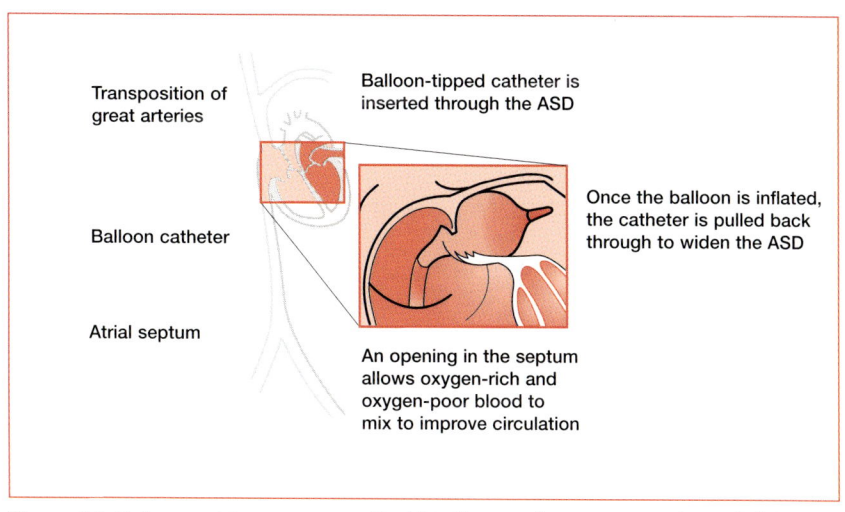

Figure 11. Balloon atrial septostomy – Rashkind's procedure. ASD: atrial septal defect.

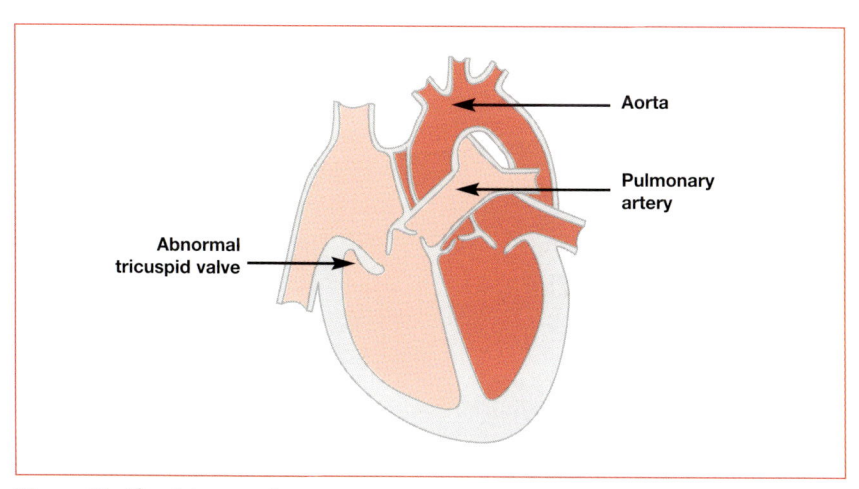

Figure 12. Ebstein's anomaly.

Chapter 14

Further reading

Deanfield J, Thaulow E, Warnes C et al.; Task Force on the Management of Grown Up Congenital Heart Disease, European Society of Cardiology; ESC Committee for Practice Guidelines. Management of grown up congenital heart disease. *Eur Heart J* 2003;24:1035–84.

Dent JM. Congenital heart disease and exercise. *Clin Sports Med* 2003;22:81–99.

Morris PJ, Wood WC, editors. *Oxford Textbook of Surgery*, 2nd edition. Oxford University Press, 2000.

Report of the British Cardiac Society Working Party. Grown-up congenital heart (GUCH) disease: current needs and provision of service for adolescents and adults with congenital heart disease in the UK. *Heart* 2002;88 (Suppl. 1):i1–14.

Abbreviations

1D	one dimensional
2D	two dimensional
A wave	atrial wave
ABPM	ambulatory blood pressure measurement
ACE	angiotensin-converting enzyme
ACEI	angiotensin-converting enzyme inhibitor
ACS	acute coronary syndromes
ADH	antidiuretic hormone
AF	atrial fibrillation
AICD	automatic implantable cardioverter defibrillator
ALT	alanine aminotransferase
ANCA	antinuclear cytoplasmic antibody
AR	aortic regurgitation
ARB	angiotensin receptor blocker
AS	aortic stenosis
ASD	atrial septal defect
AST	aspartate aminotransferase
AV	atrioventricular
AVN	atrioventricular node
AVNRT	atrioventricular nodal re-entrant tachycardia
AVR	aortic valve replacement
BP	blood pressure
bpm	beats per minute
CABG	coronary artery bypass grafting
CAD	coronary artery disease
CFM	color-flow mapping
CHD	coronary heart disease
CHF	chronic heart failure
CK-MB	creatine kinase myocardial band fraction
CNS	central nervous system
CPR	cardiopulmonary resuscitation
CRP	C-reactive protein
CT	computed tomography
CW	continuous wave
Cx	circumflex artery
CXR	chest x-ray

Abbreviations

DC	direct current
DCM	dilated cardiomyopathy
E wave	early wave
ECG	electrocardiogram
ED	erectile dysfunction
EDV	end diastolic volume
EEL	external elastic lamina
EF	ejection fraction
ESD	end systolic dimension
ESR	erythrocyte sedimentation rate
GFR	glomerular filtration rate
GP	glycoprotein
HACEK	*Haemophilus parainfluenza*, *Haemophilus aphrophilus*, *Actinobacillus (Haemophilus) actinomycetemcomitans*, *Cardiobacterium hominis*, the *Eikenella* species, and the *Kingella* species
HCM	hypertrophic cardiomyopathy
HDL	high-density lipoprotein
HIT	heparin-induced thrombocytopenia
HMG-CoA	hydroxymethylglutaryl coenzyme A
IABP	intra-aortic balloon pump
ICH	intracranial hemorrhage
ICS	intercostal space
IE	infective endocarditis
IEL	internal elastic lamina
IM	intramuscular
INR	international normalized ratio
IV	intravenous
IVC	inferior vena cava
IVDA	intravenous drug abuser
JVP	jugular venous pressure
LA	left atrium
LAD	left anterior descending artery
LBBB	left bundle branch block
LDH	lactate dehydrogenase
LDL	low-density lipoprotein
LIMA	left internal mammary artery
LLSE	left lower sternal edge
LP	lipoprotein
LP(a)	lipoprotein little a
LPL	lipoprotein lipase
LV	left ventricle
LVESD	left ventricular end-systolic dimension

Abbreviations

LVH	left ventricular hypertrophy
MET	metabolic unit
MI	myocardial infarction
MR	mitral regurgitation
MRA	magnetic resonance angiography
MRI	magnetic resonance imaging
MS	mitral stenosis
MV	mitral valve
MVA	mitral valve area
MVP	mitral valve prolapse
NYHA	New York Heart Association
PCI	percutaneous coronary intervention
PDA	persistent ductus arteriosus
PET	positron emission tomography
PTCA	percutaneous transluminal coronary angioplasty
PW	pulsed wave
QTc	corrected QT interval
RA	right atrium
RAD	right axis deviation
RBBB	right bundle branch block
RCA	right coronary artery
RIMA	right internal mammary artery
RV	right ventricle
RVH	right ventricular hypertrophy
SA	sinoatrial
SAN	sinoatrial node
SLE	systemic lupus erythematosus
SND	sinus node dysfunction
SPECT	single photon emission computed tomography
SR	sinus rhythm
SVC	superior vena cava
SVT	supraventricular tachycardia
Tc	technetium
TEE	transesophageal echocardiography
TGA	transposition of the great arteries
TIMI	Thrombosis in Myocardial Infarction
TM	tunica media
TNF	tumor necrosis factor
tPA	tissue plasminogen activator
TR	tricuspid regurgitation
VLDL	very low-density lipoprotein
VO_2 max	maximum rate of oxygen consumption

Abbreviations

VSD ventricular septal defect
VT ventricular tachycardia
WPW Wolff–Parkinson–White syndrome

Index

References to figures are in **bold**
References to tables and boxed material are in *italics*
(except where there is textual reference on the same page)

A
A waves **8**, **9**, 40
abbreviations 214–18
abciximab 64
accelerated phase hypertension 90–1
acute coronary syndromes 46
  assessment 68, **69**
  treatment 69–73
added heart sounds 11
  associations in clinical examination *12*, *13*
  relative positions **11**
adenosine challenge 125, 128
adhesion molecules 72
alanine aminotransferase (AST) 68
alpha-adrenoceptor antagonists 85, **87**
ambulatory blood pressure measurement (ABPM) 81
American Heart Association
  life-support algorithms 4
  risk factors for CAD 48
amiloride *103*
amiodarone
  arrhythmia 106, *141*, **142**
  hypertrophic cardiomyopathy 183–4
  tachycardia 72
    ventricular 128, *129*
amlodipine 54
amoxicillin/ampicillin *177*, *178*
Amplatzer occluder 207, **208**
aneurysms
  aortic 189–91
  mycotic 168
  sinus of Valsalva 191
angina 47
  pharmacological management 54–7
  silent 48
  specialist management
    assessment 57–63
    treatment 63–7
  stable 46

219

Index

symptoms 47
unstable *46*, 47
variant 48
angiotensin-converting enzyme (ACE) inhibitors
   acute coronary syndromes 72–3
   and aspirin 106
   heart failure 101, 104, *106*
   hypertension 85, 86, **87**, 88
   recommended procedure for starting *104*
angiotensin type 1 receptor blockers (ARBs)
   heart failure *106*
   hypertension 85, 86, **87**
annuloplasty 162
antiarrhythmic drugs 106, *141*, **142**
antibiotics
   infective endocarditis 173, 174–5
      prophylaxis 176, *177–8*, 207, 211
   pacemaker infection 138
   pregnancy 164
anticoagulation 54, 71, 131, **132**, 134, 156, 164
antihypertensives 82–8
   centrally-acting **86**
   mechanisms **83**
antithrombotic therapy 64
aorta **37**, **191**
aortic aneurysm 189–91
   thoracic 189, **191**
aortic dissection 191–5
   classification **192**, 193
   examination 195
   imaging **192**, **193**, **194**
   investigations 194, 195
   management 193
   presentation 194
aortic regurgitation 149–52
   acute 150
   asymptomatic patients 152
   chronic
      causes 150–1
      treatment 151–2
   common associations *12*
   echocardiography 41
   in pregnancy 164
   pulse 7
   signs 149–50
aortic root replacement 176, 193
aortic sclerosis 146
aortic stenosis
   causes 146
   common associations *12*
   echocardiography 41

Index

    investigation/management 147–9
    natural history 148
    in pregnancy 164
    pulse 7
    signs 146–7
    treatment 149
    valve replacement 148
aortic valve, bicuspid **204**, 209
aortic valve replacement (AVR) 148, 149, 151
apex beat
    abnormalities 9–10
    associations in clinical examination *12, 13*
    location 9
arrhythmia 111–43
    antiarrhythmic drugs 106, *141*, **142**
    diagnosis, possible *112*
    pulse *112*
    and thrombolysis 72
    see also specific conditions
aspartate aminotransferase (AST) 68
aspirin
    acute coronary syndromes 69
    angina 54
    atrial fibrillation 133
    chronic heart failure 106
    mitral valve prolapse 162
asthma 125
atenolol *141*
atherectomy 64
atherosclerosis *see* coronary artery disease
atrial fibrillation 130–4
    bradycardia in 118
    classification 130
    ECG **22**, 23, 130, **131**
    history *134*
    incidence/causes 130
    investigations 133
    management
        chronic 131
        new directions 134
        pharmacological 131, **132**
        surgery 134
    management of new patient 130–3
    pacing 136, *136*
    permanent 133
    presentation 130
    with pulmonary stenosis 209
    pulse 7
    in restrictive cardiomyopathy 188
atrial flutter 134
    ECG **22**, 23, **135**

Index

with pulmonary stenosis 209
atrial septal defect 205–9
    characteristics *206*
    common associations *13*
    incidence **204**
    management 207
    pathophysiology 206–7
    signs/symptoms 207
atrial tachycardia 123, **124**
atrioventricular (AV) block 117–18
    ECG **25**
    electrophysiology *141*
    first-degree 118, **119**
    second-degree *7*, 118, **119**, *136*
    third-degree (complete heart block) 118, **119**, 135, *136*
atrioventricular (AV) node **112**
atrioventricular node re-entrant tachycardia (AVNRT) 124–5
    ECG **125**
    electrophysiology *141*
    mechanisms **126**
atropine **3**, 113
auscultation 10–11
Austin Flint murmur 150
automatic implantable cardioverter defibrillator (AICD) 129, 139–40
azithromycin *32*, 177

B

balloon angioplasty 63, **65**, 209
balloon pump, intra-aortic 157
    counterpulsation 99
    insertion **99**
balloon septostomy 211, **213**
balloon valvotomy 149, 164
beating heart surgery 66
bendrofluazide 84, *87*, *103*
benzothiazepines 84
beta-agonists 94, 95, 98
beta-blockers
    acute coronary syndromes 69, 70, 72–3
    angina 54
    aortic dissection 193
    aortic regurgitation 150
    arrhythmia *141*, **142**
    atrial fibrillation 133
    heart failure 101, 104–5, *106*
    hypertension 83–4, 86, **87**, 88
    hypertrophic cardiomyopathy 183
    syncope 117
    tachyarrhythmia 123, 125
    toxicity 118
Bezold–Jarisch reflex 116, **117**

Index

bicuspid aortic valve **204**, 209
bifascicular block 121
bisferiens pulse 7
blood flow
    assessment 63, 64
    exercise-induced changes 52
    perfusion imaging 60
    velocity 36
blood pressure
    basic science 90
    guidelines 77
    heart failure 98
    measurement 78
        24-hour ambulatory 81
    see also hypertension
blood tests
    heart failure 97
    pericarditis 198
blood vessels, normal **73**
Bonet, T 102
"boot-shaped" heart 200
bounding pulse 7
bradycardia 111–19
    in atrial fibrillation 118
    atrioventricular (AV) block 117–18
        classification 118, **119**
    carotid sinus syndrome 114
    causes 113
    pacing 135, 136, *136*
    sinus node dysfunction (SND) 113–14
    syncope 114
        disturbances leading to *115*
        evaluation 114–15, *116*
        malignant vasovagal 116–17
        patterns *116*
    treatment 113
Bruce exercise protocol 57, **58**
bumetanide *103*
bundle branch block 120–2
    ECG **26**, **27**, 30, **120**
    fascicular block 120–1
    nonspecific intraventricular conduction defect 122
bundle of His 18, **112**, 120, **121**
bundle of Kent 125–7
bupropion 49
"butterfly" occluding devices 207, **208**

C

cachexia 5
CAD *see* coronary artery disease
caffeine and hypertension 78, 82

Index

calcification, valve **153**
calcium-channel blockers
    acute coronary syndromes 73
    angina 54
    aortic dissection 193
    atrial fibrillation 133
    hypertension 84, 87, 88
    hypertrophic cardiomyopathy 183
    toxicity 118
calcium levels
    in atherosclerotic plaque 62
    hypertension 80
calcium sensitizers 106
captopril 101
carcinoid syndrome 188
cardiac arrest
    causes 2, 3
    electrophysiology *141*
    life-support algorithms *1–3*
cardiac catheterization 63–6, 69
    aortic stenosis 149
    complications 65
    history *63*
    hypertrophic cardiomyopathy 184
    mortality 66
cardiac markers *see* markers
cardiac rehabilitation 74, 75
cardiac resynchronization therapy (CRT) 107
cardiac tamponade 199–200
    examination 199–200
    imaging 200
    pulse *7*
cardiogenic shock
    management **99**
    and PTCA 70
cardiomegaly **98**
cardiomyopathy *see* dilated cardiomyopathy; hypertrophic cardiomyopathy; restrictive cardiomyopathy
cardiopulmonary resuscitation (CPR) 2, 3
cardiovascular examinations *see* examinations, cardiovascular
cardioversion
    chemical 133
    direct current (DC) 127, 133, 134
    implantable cardioverter defibrillators 139–40
    spontaneous 130–1
carotid sinus massage 124
carotid sinus syndrome 114, *136*
catheterization *see* cardiac catheterization
cefadroxil *177*
cefazolin *177*
cephalexin *177*

Index

chemokines 52, 72
chest leads *see under* electrocardiography
chest pain
    atypical 47
    differentiation 47
    investigations 53
    likelihood of CAD 59
chest X-ray
    aortic dissection **194**
    cardiac tamponade 200
    cardiomegaly **98**
    coronary artery disease 54
    dilated cardiomyopathy 187
    heart failure 93, 96, **97**, **98**
    pericarditis 198
    pleural effusion **97**, **98**
    pulmonary stenosis 210
    ventricular septal defect 204
cholesterol
    and coronary artery disease 52
    as risk factor 48, 49, *50–1*
    synthesis/transport 55, **56**
cholestyramine 56
chronotropic incompetence 136
chylomicrons 55, **56**
Clamshell occluder 207, **208**
clarithromycin 32, 177
clindamycin 32, 177
cloxacillin (flucloxacillin) 138, 175
clonidine 85, **86**
clopidogrel 54, 64, 69
cloxacillin (flucloxacillin) 138, 175
clubbing 5, 6, 167, 203, 210
coarctation of aorta 172, **204**, 209
collapsing pulse 7
complete heart block 118, **119**, 135, *136*
computed tomography (CT) **192**
congenital bicuspid disease 164
congenital heart disease 203–14
    atrial septal defect 13, **204**, 205–9
    bicuspid aortic valve **204**
    children 203
    coarctation of aorta 172, **204**, 209
    Ebstein's anomaly 162, 211, **213**
    Fallot's tetralogy **204**, 210, **212**
    patent ductus arteriosus 7, 13, **204**, 210
    pulmonary stenosis 13, **204**, 209–10
    right bundle branch block 203
    signs 6, 203
    transposition of the great arteries **204**, 210–11, **212**
    ventricular septal defect 13, 157, 172, 203–5
Conn's syndrome 80

225

Index

constrictive pericarditis 200–1
contractile proteins 181, **182**
contrast echocardiography 38–9
corneal arcus 6
coronary angiography (the first example of) 66
coronary artery bypass grafting (CABG) 66, **67**
coronary artery disease (atherosclerosis) 45–76, 189, 191
   assessment 47–8
   background 45–6
   diagnostic algorithm 59, **61**
   door-to-needle time 53
   initiation 72
   investigations 53–4
   management 48–57
   pharmacological management 54–7
   presentations 46
   risk factors 48–53
      American Heart Association 48
      European Society of Cardiology 49
      risk estimation 53
      risk tables 50–1, 53
   specialist management
      assessment 57–63
      evidence base 67
      treatment 63–7
   see also acute coronary syndromes; angina
Corrigan's sign 149
cotrimoxazole 175
Coumadin *see* warfarin
creatine kinase 68, **69**
creatine kinase myocardial band fraction (CKMB) 68, **69**
cyanosis 203, 210
cyanotic heart disease 172, 210

D

de Musset, A 161
de Musset's sign 149
depolarization 18, **20**
diabetes 48, 51, 88
   therapy 72
diastolic dysfunction 40
diet 52, 75, 82
digoxin/digitalis 107
   atrial fibrillation 133
   heart failure 105, 106
   mechanism of action **105**
   toxicity 30, 118
dihydropyridines 54, 73, 84
dilated cardiomyopathy 186–7
diltiazem
   acute coronary syndromes 69

Index

angina 54
aortic dissection 193
arrhythmia *141*
hypertension 84, 86
dimensions, intracardiac *39*
disopyramide 117, 129, *141*
diuretics
    heart failure **102**, *103*
    hypertension 84, **87**, 88
diving reflex 125
dobutamine 60, 107, 150, 157, 184
dopamine 150
Doppler imaging 36–8
    aortic stenosis 147–9
    atrial septal defect **206**
    color-flow mapping 38
    continuous-wave 37
    normal values *39*
    pulsed-wave 37, 40
doxazosin 85, 87
doxycycline 175
Dressler's syndrome 198
drug abuse, intravenous 162, 169, 175
drug-eluting stents 63
drug-induced abnormalities of ECG 29, *30*, *32*
drug toxicity 118
Duchenne de Boulogne, GBA *24*
Duke criteria *170*
Duke risk score **60**
Duroziez's sign 149
dyspnea 48, 95, 108
    acute nocturnal 95
    after exercise 210

E

E waves 40
E:A ratios *39*, 40
Ebstein's anomaly 162, 211, **213**
echocardiography 35–43
    aortic dissection **193**
    aortic stenosis 147–9
    applications 39–42
    atrial septal defect **206**
    background 35
    cardiac tamponade 200
    contrast 38–9
    dilated cardiomyopathy 187
    EF measurements 100
    fractional shortening 39
    heart failure 93, 97, 100
    hypertrophic cardiomyopathy 183

Index

imaging modes 35–8
  see also M-mode imaging; two-dimensional imaging
infective endocarditis 42, 174, 175
mitral regurgitation 157
mitral stenosis 155
mitral valve vegetation 158, 172
normal values 39
pericarditis 198
restrictive cardiomyopathy 187–8
syncope 115
transesophageal (TEE) 38
views 35, **36**
  see also stress echocardiography
Einthoven, W 25
Eisenmenger syndrome 207, 210
ejection click 11, *147*, 210
elderly patients
  aortic stenosis 146
  hypertension 87–8
  valve replacement 149
electrocardiography (ECG) 15–33
  aortic stenosis 146
  atrial fibrillation **131**
  atrial flutter **135**
  atrial tachycardia **124**
  AV block **119**
  AV re-entrant tachycardia **125**
  axis calculation 22–3
  bundle branch block **120**
  cardiac tamponade 200
  carrying out 15
  coronary artery disease 53–4
  discovery 25
  electrophysiological studies 140, *141*, 142
  exercise ECG *see* exercise electrocardiography
  general principles 15, 16
  heart failure 96
  history
    discovery 25
    dog demonstrating ECG 18
    first resuscitation 24
    lettering system 33
  hypertrophic cardiomyopathy 183
  interpretation 21–2
  leads
    attachment sites **16**
    chest 17, **20**
    definitions 15
    limb 16, **17**
    respective views of heart *17*
  left axis deviation **122**

228

Index

mitral stenosis **155**
pacemakers 139
pericarditis 198
planes of view 17
pulmonary stenosis 210
rate/rhythm 22
restrictive cardiomyopathy 187
right axis deviation **123**
syncope 114–15
trace 19–23
    basic pattern **19**
    drug-induced abnormalities 29
    lettering system *33*
    normal **21**
    pattern combinations 30
    see also specific segments/waves
    variations
        normal 24
        pathological 25–33
    ventricular septal defect 204
    wave direction/size 21
see also exercise electrocardiography
electron beam computed tomography 62
electrophysiological studies 140–1
    indications *141*
embolism sources, cardiac 42
end-organ damage in hypertension 80
endocarditis *see* infective endocarditis
endomyocardial fibrosis 188
endothelin antagonists 106
energy-related proteins 181
enterococci *170*, 171
eosinophilic cardiomyopathy 188
eptifibatide 64
erectile dysfunction 88–9
esmolol 125
European Society of Cardiology
    risk factors for cardiovascular disease 78
    risk factors for coronary artery disease 49
examinations, cardiovascular 5–14, 47
    auscultation 10–11
    general inspection 5
    jugular venous pressure 7–9
    palpation 9–10
    pulse 5–6
exercise
    in angina 53
    in aortic regurgitation 152
    beneficial effects 52–3
    cardiac rehabilitation 75
    and chest pain 47

Index

Fallot's tetralogy 210
   and hypertension 82
   ventricular ectopics in 129
exercise electrocardiography 57
   contraindications 59
   interpretation 58
   pretest likelihood of disease 58, **59**
   stable angina 57–9
   stopping, reasons for 59
exercise testing 115, 149, 151
   with gas analysis 100
exercise training 106

F

facial signs 6
Fallot's tetralogy 210, **212**
   incidence **204**
fascicular block 120–1
fatty acid binding proteins as markers 68
fibrates 56
first-degree AV block 118, **119**
flecainide 30, 129, 131, 133, *141*, **142**
Forssmann, W 63
Framingham risk tables 78
Frank–Starling curve **95**, **159**
Friedrich's sign 199
fungal infections 171, 175
furosemide (frusemide) 98, *103*

G

genetic disorders 5
gentamicin 175, *178*
Goswell, T **18**
GPIIb/IIIa inhibitors
   acute coronary syndromes 69, 70, 71
   angina 64

H

HACEK organisms *170*, 171, 173
"hardening of arteries" 45, 47
heart block *see* atrioventricular (AV) block
heart failure 93–109
   background 93
   causes 93
   chronic **96**
      diagnosis/assessment 100
      nonpharmacological treatment 106–8
      pharmacological treatment 100–1, 104–6
   examination/clinical history 95
   history *102*
   investigations 96–7

Index

management **102**, *103*
  acute heart failure 98
  chronic heart failure 100–1, 104–6
  future directions 106
  history *107*
  by NYHA classification *106*
  palliative care 108
  pathophysiology 94–5
  with pulmonary stenosis 209
  symptoms, multiorgan *94*
  systolic vs diastolic 93
  treatment **95**
heart fatty-acid binding proteins 68
heart murmur
  asymptomatic 145–6
  grading *145*
heart sounds 10–11
  added 11, *12, 13*
  aortic regurgitation 150
  aortic stenosis 149
  associations in clinical examination *12, 13*
  atrial septal defect 207
  cardiac tamponade 199
  congenital heart disease 203
  mitral regurgitation *154*, 159
  mitral stenosis 154, *155*
  mitral valve prolapse 161
  patent ductus arteriosus 210
  pericarditis 198
  physiological splitting 10
  pulmonary stenosis 209–10
  relative positions **11**
  ventricular septal defect 204
heart "wiring" **112**
Heberden, W 47
heparin 69, 70–1, 164
Herrick, JA 45
hibernating myocardium 62
high-density lipoprotein (HDL) 48, *49*, 53, 55–57
history-taking 47, 78
Holter monitoring 114–15
homocystinuria 87, 191
Hopps, J *137*
hydralazine
  heart failure 105, *106*
  hypertension 85, 88
hydrochlorothiazide 87, *103*
hyperaldosteronism 80
hyperkalemia 30, **31**
hyperlipidemia 6, 55–6
hypertension 77–91

Index

assessment
  examination 79–80
  history-taking 78
  investigations 80–1, 89
background 77
basic science 90
blood pressure guidelines 77
causes 78, 79
definition 77–8
malignant/accelerated phase 90–1
management
  generalist 89
  lifestyle changes 81–2
  pharmacotherapy 82–7
  special populations 87–9
resistant 81, 90
symptoms 78
systolic vs diastolic 86–7
hypertensive retinopathy 81
hypertrophic cardiomyopathy (HCM) 181–6
  background 181–2
  echocardiography 42
  examinations 183
  management
    medical 183–4
    nonsurgical septal reduction 184
    pacing 184
    surgery 184–5
  mutations causing 181, 182
  nonobstructive 186
  pulse 7
  screening before sport 185–6

I

imidazoline type 1 receptor agonists 85, **86**
infective endocarditis
  causative organisms 169–71, 175
  diagnostic classification 169, 170
  echocardiography 42, 174, 175
  investigations 173–4
  location 162
  and mitral regurgitation 159
  pathogenesis 172
  prognosis 176
  prophylaxis 176, 177–8, 207, 211
  prosthetic valves 172–3
  referral 173
  signs 6, 167
  symptoms 167–9
    constitutional 167
    eyes 168

 neurological 168
 renal 168
 skin lesions 167
 treatment
  antibiotics 173, 174–5
  surgical 175–6
 and ventricular septal defect 204, 205
inflammation in atherosclerosis 72
inotropes 72, 94, 95
intra-aortic balloon pump
 counterpulsation 99
 insertion **99**
 in mitral regurgitation 157
intracranial hemorrhage (ICH) 70
irregularly irregular pulse 7
isoproterenol (isoprenaline) 113
isotopes in CAD assessment 59, 60

J
Janeway lesions 6, 167, *170*
Jenner, E 47
Jervell and Lange-Nielsen syndrome *30*, 130
"jet" lesions 159, 172
jugular veins **9**
jugular venous pressure (JVP) 7–9
 abnormalities *9*
 associations in clinical examination *12*, *13*
 positioning 8, **9**
 waveforms **8**

K
Kavanagh, T 74
Kussmaul, A *200*
Kussmaul breathing *200*
Kussmaul's sign 199, *200*

L
labetalol 88, 91, 193
lactate dehydrogenase *68*, **69**
Laennec *148*
left anterior/posterior fascicular block 121
left bundle branch **112**
left bundle branch block (LBBB)
 ECG **26**, **27**, 120
 hypertrophic cardiomyopathy 183
left ventricular hypertrophy
 ECG **26**, 29
 with hypertension 80–1
 and hypertrophic cardiomyopathy 181
left ventricular mass in HCM **183**
lidocaine (lignocaine)

233

Index

arrhythmia *141*, **142**
　ventricular tachycardia 128
life-support algorithms for cardiac arrest
　advanced UK 2, *4*
　advanced US 3, *4*
　basic adult *1*, *4*
lifestyle changes
　acute coronary syndromes 74
　and hypertension 81–2
limb leads *see under* electrocardiography
Lincoln, A *190*
lipid-lowering agents 55–7
lipid transport 55, **56**
lipoproteins 55–56
loop diuretics 84
　heart failure 98, *103*
low-density lipoprotein (LDL) *48*, *49*, 55–57, 72

M

M-mode imaging 36, **37**
Mackenzie, J *134*
macrophage foam cells **46**, 72
magnesium
　in ventricular tachycardia 72, 128
　in pregnancy 88
magnetic resonance angiography (MRA) 62–3
magnetic resonance imaging (MRI)
　angina 62–3
　aortic dissection **192**
　pacemakers 139
malar flush 6
malignant hypertension 90–1
malignant vasovagal syncope 116–17
　pacing *136*
Marfan's syndrome 5, 189, *190*, 191
markers
　inflammation 72
　myocardial damage *68*, **69**
Maze procedure 134
methyldopa 85, **86**, 88
metolazone 101, *103*
metoprolol 101, 131
microbubbles 38–9
minoxidil 85
mitral regurgitation 157–60
　acute 157–8
　asymptomatic patients 159–60
　causes *154*, 158, 160
　chronic 158–60
　common associations *12*
　echocardiography 41

functional 160
  natural history 159
  in pregnancy 164
  signs *154, 158*, 159
  therapy 160
mitral stenosis 152–7
  and atrial fibrillation 156–7
  causes 152, *154*
  common associations *12*
  echocardiography 41, *42*, **155**
  ECG **155**
  left atrial dilatation **154**
  in pregnancy 164
  signs 6, 153–4, 155
  therapy **155**
    medical 156
    surgical 155–6
mitral valve apparatus **153**
mitral valves
  echocardiography **37**
  prolapse 42, 161–2
  repair/replacement *156*
  vegetation **158, 172**
Mobitz I (Wenckebach) AV block 118, **119**
Mobitz II AV block 118, **119**
  pacing *136*
Morgagni, G 47
morphine 108
Morrow procedure 184
Müller's sign 150
murmurs 11
  adult congenital heart disease 203
  aortic regurgitation *147*, 149–150
  aortic stenosis 147
  associations in clinical examination *12, 13*
  asymptomatic 145–146
  atrial septal defect 206, 207
  hypertrophic cardiomyopathy 183
  infective endocarditis 167, *170*
  mitral regurgitation *154*, 157, *158*, 159
  mitral stenosis *154, 155*
  mitral valve prolapse 161
  patent ductus arteriosus 210
  in pregnancy 163
  preparticipation screening in sport *185*
  pulmonary valve disease 163
  pulmonary valve stenosis 210
  tricuspid valve disease 162
  ventricular septal defect 204, *206*
Mustard operation 211
mycotic aneurysms 168

Index

myocardial fiber disarray 182
myocardial infarction (MI) 46
   in acute coronary syndromes 70
   acute, definition of 46
   anteroseptal 27
   ECG 25, **27**
   thrombosis in 45
myoglobin 68, **69**

N
natriuretic peptides 97
neutral endopeptidase inhibitors 106
nicorandil 55
nifedipine 152
nitrates
   acute coronary syndromes 69
   angina 54
   heart failure 98, 105, *106*
nitric oxide 52
nitroprusside 91, 150, 157
nonspecific intraventricular conduction defect 122
nuclear cardiology 59–61

O
opiates 69, 108
orthopnea 95
Osler, W *171*
Osler's nodes 6, 167, **168**, *170*
ostium primum/secundum 205, 207
oxygen therapy 69

P
P waves 19, 22
   abnormalities 30
   atrial tachycardia 123
pacemaker syndrome 138
pacemakers 135–40
   AAI 136
   automatic implantable cardioverter defibrillator (AICD) 139–40
   avoidance of magnetic fields 139
   codes 135–6, *137*
   complications 138–9
   DDD 118, 121, 135–6, 138, 184
   DDI 114
   ECG 139
   first artificial 24
   history *137*
   implantation 137–8
   indications, standard *136*
   mode switching 138
   patient follow-up 139

Index

permanent dual-chamber 114, 123
program alteration 138
rate-adaptive 136
single lead atrial 114
testing 137
VVI 136, 138
pacing
   atrial fibrillation 136
   atrial tachycardia 123
   atrioventricular (AV) block 118, 135, *136*
   bifascicular block 121
   bradycardia 114, 135, 136
      external 113
   hypertrophic cardiomyopathy 184
   sinus node dysfunction *136*
   syncope *136*
   trifascicular block 121
palpation 9–10
papillary muscle dysfunction 157, 160
paraprosthetic regurgitation 42
Parry, C 47
patent ductus arteriosus 210, **211**
   common associations 13
   incidence **204**
   pulse 7
patent foramen ovale 210
patient education in chronic heart failure 100–1
percutaneous techniques 63, 64–6
   balloon aortic valvotomy 149
   balloon mitral valvotomy 164
   evidence base 67
   valvotomy 155–6
percutaneous transluminal coronary angioplasty (PTCA) 63, 70
perfusion imaging 59–61
pericardial disease 197–201
   cardiac tamponade 199–200
   pericardial effusion 199
   pericarditis 197–9
      constrictive 200–1
pericardial effusion 199
pericarditis 197–9
   causes *198*
   constrictive 200–1
   ECG 29
   examination 198
   imaging 198
   investigations 198
   management 199
   pathophysiology 197
   presentations 198
pericardium **197**

Index

petechiae 167
phenylalkylamine derivatives 84
physical activity *see* exercise
pipercillin 175
pitting edema 5
plaques, coronary
    formation 72
    range 45
    ruptured 45, **46**
    stable 45, **46**
    unstable 45, **46**
pleural effusion **97**
potassium blood levels 80, 97
potassium-channel openers 55
potassium-sparing diuretics *103*, *104*
PR interval 19
    abnormalities 30
prazosin 85, *87*
pregnancy and hypertension 88
procainamide *141*
propafenone *32*, 129, *141*
proptosis 6
prostacyclin 52
prosthetic valve endocarditis 173, 174
prothrombotic factors 45
pulmonary edema 95, *102*
pulmonary embolism 30
pulmonary hypertension *13*, 207
pulmonary regurgitation *12*
pulmonary stenosis *13*, **204**, 209–10
pulmonary valve disease 163
pulses 5–7
    abnormal 7
    associations in clinical examination *12*, *13*
    peripheral 6
pulsus alternans 7
pulsus paradoxus *7*, *200*
Purkinje system 18

Q

Q waves **25**, 26
QRS wave complex 19, 20, 22, **25**
    abnormalities **27**, 30, **31**
    large/broad 27
    sinus wave 30, **33**
    Wolff–Parkinson–White syndrome 126
QT interval
    abnormalities 29, *30*
        drug-induced 29, *30*, *32*
    torsade de pointes 129–30
Quincke's sign 150

quinidine *141*, **142**

R
radioactive stents 64
radiofemoral delay 80
radiofrequency ablation
    atrial flutter 134
    tachyarrhythmia 123, 125
    Wolff–Parkinson–White syndrome *127*
Rashkind's procedure 211, **213**
recanalization 71
referral
    acute coronary syndromes 73
    aortic stenosis 146
    coronary artery disease 57
    hypertension 89
regularly irregular pulse 7
renin–angiotensin system antagonists 85
resistant hypertension 81, 90
restrictive cardiomyopathy 187–8
Resuscitation Council (UK) 4
resuscitation, first electrical 24
retinopathy, hypertensive 80
revascularization 107
rheumatic heart disease 152, 162, 172
rifampicin 175
right bundle branch **112**
right bundle branch block (RBBB)
    and congenital heart disease 203
    ECG **27**, 30, 120
right ventricular hypertrophy **27**
risk estimation of coronary artery disease 53
risk tables
    coronary artery disease *50–1*, 53
    and hypertension 78
Romano–Ward syndrome *30*, 130
Roth spots 168, *170*

S
saphenous vein graft 66, **67**
sawtooth P waves 23
scavenger receptors 72
second-degree AV block 118, **119**
secondary hypertension 79
sick sinus syndrome *see* sinus node dysfunction
sildenafil 89
single photon emission computed tomography (SPECT) 60
sinoatrial node (SAN) 18, **112**
sinus node dysfunction (sick sinus syndrome) 113–14, *136*, *141*
sinus of Valsalva, aneurysm of 191
sinus tachycardia 123

Index

sinus venosus **206**
smoking
   cessation 49, 82
   as risk factor 48, 49, *50–1*
sodium levels
   heart failure 97
   hypertension 80
Sokolow–Lyon index 27
sotalol *30*, *32*, 129, *141*, **142**, 184
specialist nursing 108
spironolactone 83, 101, **102**, *103*, *104*, *106*
splinter hemorrhages 6, 167, 168
spondyloarthritides 5
ST segment 21
   abnormalities **27**, 28–9
   diagnostic exercise tests 57–8
   elevation in acute coronary syndromes 70
   reverse tick depression 30
staphylococci *170*, 171
Starflex occluder 207
statins 56, 57
stents 63, **65**, 67
stethoscope, invention of *148*
Stokes–Adams attacks 118
"strain" **26**, 29, 30
streptococci 169, *170*
streptokinase 70–1
stress echocardiography 61–2
stunned atria 133
stunned myocardium 62
"swinging heart" **199**
sympathomimetics 85
syncope 114
   disturbances leading to *115*
   electrophysiology *141*
   evaluation 114–15, *116*
   malignant vasovagal 116–17
   pacing *136*
   patterns *116*
syndrome X 48
systolic dysfunction 40

T

T waves 21
   abnormalities **26**, 29, 30
   inversion **28**
tachyarrhythmia 122–34
   atrial fibrillation 130–4
   atrial flutter 134
   atrial tachycardia 123, **124**
   AV node re-entrant tachycardia (AVNRT) 124–5, **126**

diagnosis 122, *124*
ECG 122
sinus tachycardia 123
torsade de pointes 129–30
ventricular ectopics 129
ventricular pre-excitation 125–7
ventricular tachycardia 128–9
tachycardia–bradycardia syndrome *see* sinus node dysfunction
teeth 5
teicoplanin 175
thiazide diuretics
heart failure *103*
hypertension 84, 86, 87, 88
third-degree AV block (complete heart block) 118, **119**, 135, *136*
three-vessel disease 66
thrombolysis 70
acute coronary syndromes 70–1
arrhythmia 72
complications 70
contraindications 71
recanalization after 71
thrombosis 45, **46**
thyroid problems 80
ticlopidine 64
tilt-table testing 117
TIMI (Thrombolysis in Myocardial Infarction) 63, *64*
tirofiban 64
tissue plasminogen activator (tPA) 70, 71
TNF-α antibodies 106
torasemide *103*
torsades de pointes 32, 129–30
transesophageal echocardiography (TEE) 38, 174
transplantation 107–8
transposition of the great arteries **204**, 210–11, **212**
transthoracic two-dimensional echocardiography 174
Traube's sign 150
triamterene *103*
tricuspid valve disorders
Ebstein's anomaly 162, 211, **213**
regurgitation 12
stenosis 13
tricuspid valve replacement 162
trifascicular block 121
triglycerides 55
troponins 46, 64, 68, 69, 70, 181, **182**
Twiddler's syndrome 138
two-dimensional imaging 35, **36**

U
ultrasound 35
see also echocardiography; stress echocardiography

Index

V

vagolytics 117
Valsalva maneuver 124
valve assessment 41
valve disease 145–65
    aortic regurgitation 149–52
    aortic stenosis 146–9
    heart murmur 145–6
    mitral regurgitation 157–60
    mitral stenosis 152–7
    mitral valve prolapse 161–2
    in pregnancy 163–4
    pulmonary 163
    tricuspid 162–3
valve replacement
    aortic (AVR) 148, 149, 151, 193
    in endocarditis 176
    tricuspid 162
vancomycin 175, *178*
vasoconstrictive factors 45
vasodilators 60, 85, 95, 105, 152, 164
Vaughan-Williams classification *141*
vector diagram of QRS axis 23
vegetations
    infective endocarditis 172, 173, 204
    mitral valves **158**, 159
ventricular assist devices 107–8
ventricular dysynchrony 107
ventricular ectopics (premature beats) 129
ventricular hypertrophy
    left **26**, 29
    right **27**
ventricular pre-excitation 125–7
ventricular septal defect 157, 172, 203–5
    characteristics *206*
    common associations *13*
    incidence **204**
ventricular tachycardia 128–9
    chronic 129
    ECG 128
    polymorphic vs monomorphic 129
ventriculography 60, 61
verapamil
    angina 54
    aortic dissection 193
    arrhythmia *141*
    hypertension 84, 86
    hypertrophic cardiomyopathy 183
    tachyarrhythmia 125
viral pericarditis 198

Index

W
wall-motion abnormality 40–1
Waller, AD **18**, 25
warfarin
 acute coronary syndromes 73
 angina 54
 atrial fibrillation 131, 133
 mitral valve prolapse 162
 in pregnancy 164
waterhammer pulse 7, 149
weight reduction 75, 82
Welch, H *102*
Wenckebach (Mobitz I) AV block 118, **119**
Withering, W *107*
Wolff–Parkinson–White (WPW) syndrome 125–6
 ECG 127
 electrophysiology *141*
 history *127*

X
xanthomata 6

Z
Zyban 49